Authored by Nicholas D Carignan
Photography by Anna Gatt
First Edition 2025

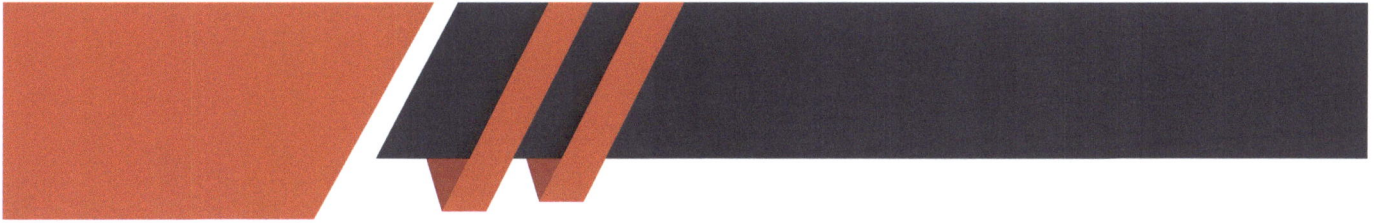

Stronger On Scene

A 45-Day Blueprint for Strength & Stamina for First Responders

Authored by Nicholas D Carignan

Dedication

To my wife, Monica, and our kids who are the driving force behind my motivation to return home safely after every shift.

To all the men and women who have dedicated their careers to facing the unknown, serving the unseen, and protecting the greater good of humanity.

Table of Content

Stronger On Scene

Disclaimer

There are significant risks involved in all aspects of physical training. These risks include but are not limited to: falls which can result in serious injury or death; injury or death due to negligence on the part of yourself, your training partner, or other people around you; injury or death due to improper use or failure of equipment; strains and sprains. Neither this training program nor any other training program should be followed without first consulting a health care professional. Individual results from this training program or any training program will vary from person to person. The author and publisher make no guarantee or warranty regarding anyone person's individual results from utilizing the training program contained herein.

The author and publisher specifically disclaim any liability, loss or risk, personal or otherwise, which is incurred as a consequence, directly or indirectly, of the use and application of any of the contents of this book. Furthermore, those following this training program willingly assume full responsibility for the risks that they are exposing themselves to and accept full responsibility for any injury or death that may result from participation in any activity described herein.

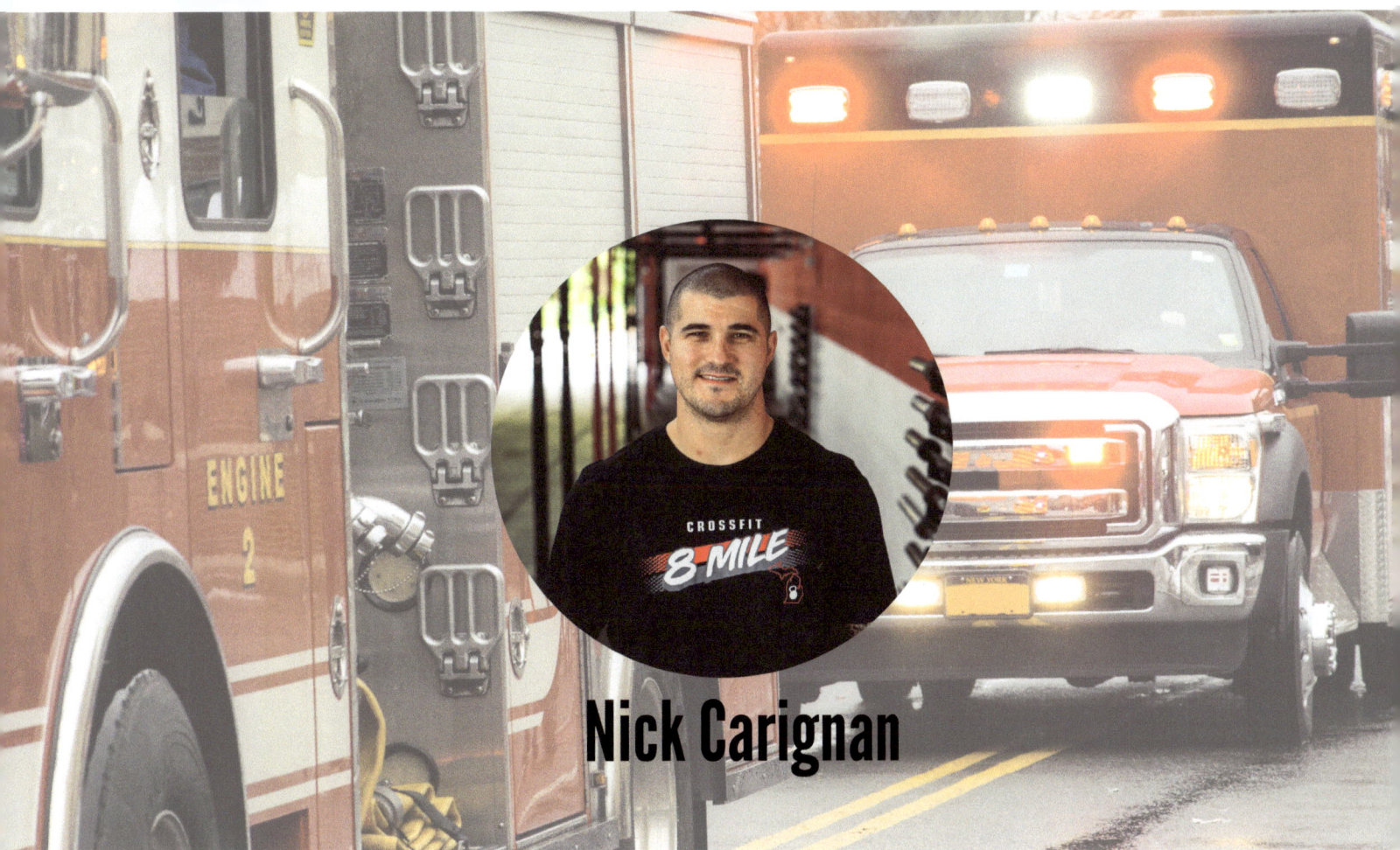

Nick Carignan

My name is Nick Carignan, and I'm a second-generation firefighter and paramedic. For the past 17 years, I've served as a professional firefighter and paramedic while also dedicating the last 15 years to coaching strength and conditioning. Owning and operating my own training facility has given me the freedom to refine my approach to fitness—one that goes beyond traditional lifting and into functional, job-specific conditioning.

When I first joined the fire service, I was a classic gym rat—hitting traditional muscle group splits, lifting heavy, and power-walking past the cardio machines like they didn't exist. I was strong, but I wasn't necessarily prepared for the demands of the job. It didn't take long to realize that real-world performance required more than just muscle—it required endurance, durability, and the ability to work under extreme fatigue.

That realization led me to explore new training methods. I fell in love with CrossFit for its blend of strength and conditioning, but over time, my focus evolved into a more kettlebell-centric, gritty, and practical approach—one built around the reality of the job.

Stronger On Scene

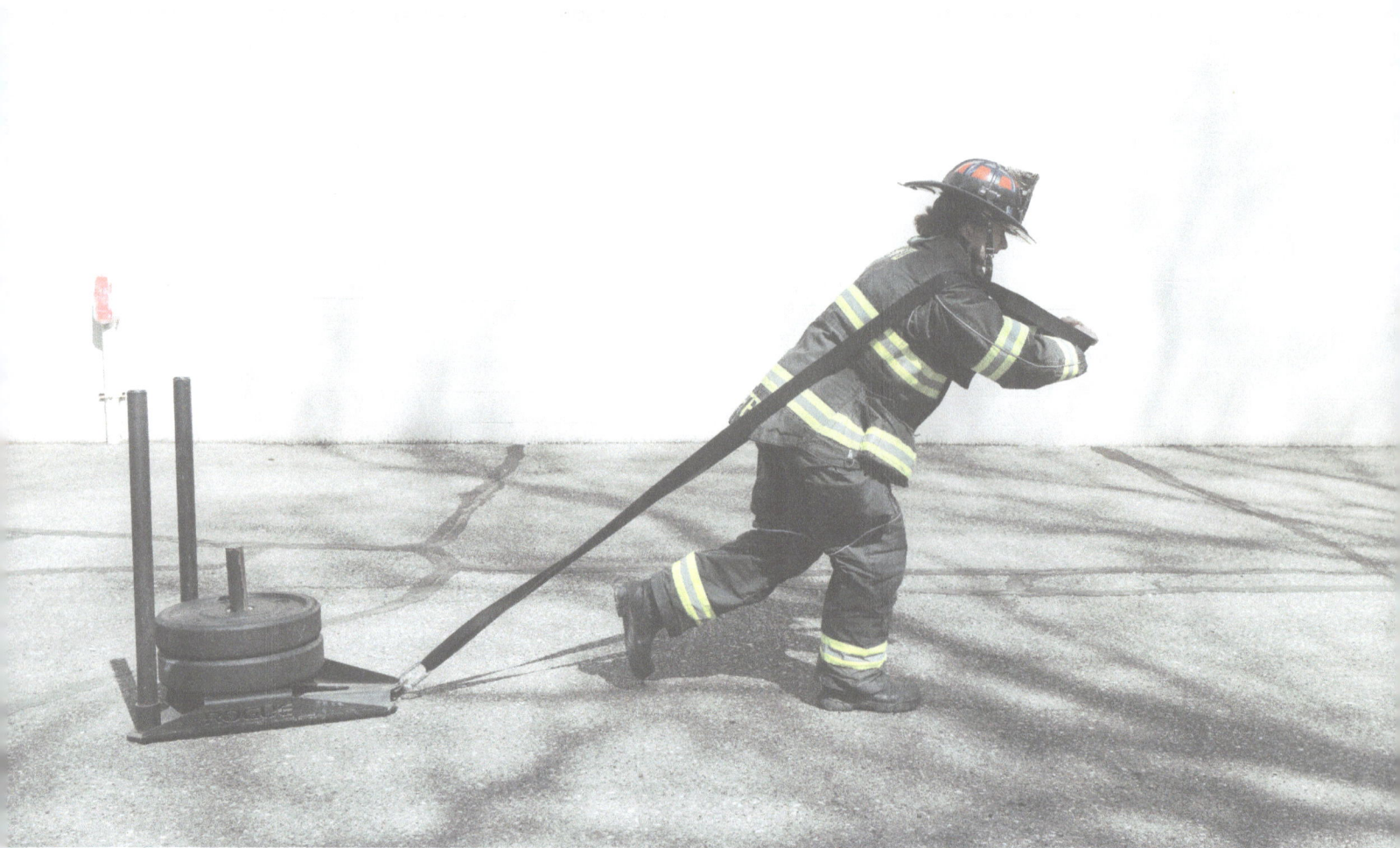

Why This Program?

As first responders, we don't need to be the fastest or the strongest in a traditional sense. What we do need is the ability to be strong under fatigue, to endure, and to perform when it matters most. We don't get to choose when the call comes or how long the job will last—our training should reflect that reality.

This program is designed to prepare you for the unpredictable nature of the job. It's about building strength, resilience, and the capacity to perform in high-stress, physically demanding situations. Whether you're pulling a charged hose line, carrying a patient down a flight of stairs, or working a long scene in full gear, this training will help ensure that when the moment comes, you're ready.

Each training day is carefully calculated based on what came before and what's coming next. The progression is intentional—designed to build strength, resilience, and skill over time. Skipping ahead or bouncing around disrupts that rhythm and can stall your progress. Stay the path, trust the process, and you'll move forward. Resist the urge to chase the shiny object—real growth comes from consistency, not novelty.

Practicality Matters

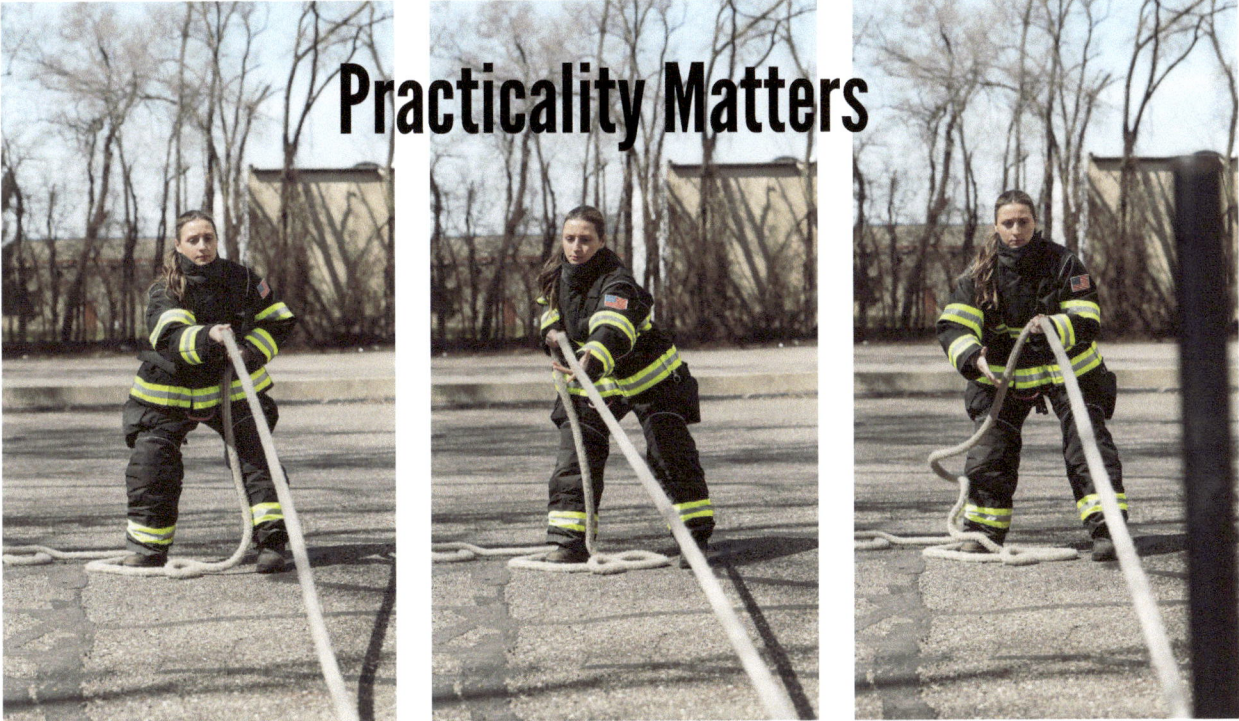

As first responders, we don't get to choose the time, place, duration, or intensity of the challenges we face. The demands are unpredictable, and training for a moving target requires an approach that is broad, adaptable, and powerful. Strength, cardiovascular endurance, and multi-directional movement aren't optional—they're essential.

Relying solely on machines for strength training and separating cardio into another session won't cut it. To perform at your best—whether as a firefighter, law enforcement officer, emergency medical personnel, or military professional—you need to train dynamically, integrating strength, endurance, and movement in every plane.

This program is built for that purpose. With a structured training plan that varies in modality, intensity, load, and style, it ensures balanced progress while preventing burnout and injury. The key to success isn't just intensity—it's consistency. Show up, put in the work, and become the best responder you can be.

What's Your Why?

After training countless cadets through the fire academy, I've seen every type of person walk through those doors—different backgrounds, shapes, sizes, and levels of physical preparedness. Some came ready. Many did not. And every time, I ask the same question:

"What did you think you were signing up for?"

Because let's be real—this isn't a job. It's a calling.
It's physical. It's mental. It's emotional.

Even when it's glorified in movies or hyped on social media—it's still action. Always.

So why did you choose this path?
Why fire? Why police? Why EMS? Why military?
Because these professions are hard. And they're meant to be. They demand the best of you on your worst days.

And I'm not just talking about on shift.
I'm talking about the grind **off shift**—when you're trying to squeeze in training between missed sleep, missed birthdays, missed moments. When you're constantly playing catch-up with the rest of your life.

If you joined for the glory, you're going to get exposed.
Because **your "why" has to be bigger than you.**

Training isn't about looking good. It's about **being good**—at your job, in the moment, under pressure.

It's about being an **asset,** not a liability.

It's about your officer having confidence that when they say, "Go," you deliver—no hesitation.

Stronger On Scene

Your training is the edge that lets you walk into a fire, a domestic, or a cardiac arrest call with calm readiness—not panic.

Because here's the hard truth:
"I'm out of shape" is not a valid excuse to a grieving family.
"I didn't have it today" doesn't fly when someone's life was on the line.
"I wasn't strong enough" won't comfort your partner's spouse if you couldn't pull them out.

Being physically incapable is **not an excuse**—not in this line of work.
There are countless things you can't control on scene.
But **your fitness?** That's 100% within your grasp.
Your **workouts**, your **diet**, your **physical preparedness**—all in your hands.

This job will wear you down. That's a fact. But the stronger you are—body and mind—the more you can carry. The more years you'll last. And the more likely you are to walk away with your health and your purpose intact.

You don't have to be the strongest.
You don't have to be the fastest.
But you damn sure have to be able to operate at 80-85% output—for hours, if needed.

That's the reality. Some days you'll have more in the tank, some less. But if you train with consistency, that 80-85% will always be there. **Ready. Reliable. Relentless.**

Long-term consistency beats short-term intensity—every time.
The real ones? They don't show up once.
They show up **again. And again. And again.**
At the same level. Or higher.
That's where the real ones are built.

So I'll ask you again—
What's your why?

The Importance of Rest Days

Being a first responder can fuel the adrenaline junkie in us, but it also brings restless nights, full moons, and back-to-back rescue calls. The job takes a toll—not just physically, but on our nervous system and hormones as well. While staying fit and active is essential for the demands of our profession, prioritizing rest and recovery is just as crucial.

Early in my career, working low on the seniority list, I treated shift days as either rest days or a chance to squeeze in a workout before the madness began. Once the shift started, training became a gamble—sometimes possible, often not. The unpredictability of EMS means you never know what the night will bring, making it tough to plan training for the following day.

If you're feeling drained and struggling to keep up, listen to your body. Take a rest day. Grab a nap and try to train later, or push your session to tomorrow. Recovery isn't weakness—it's part of longevity in this career.

That said, we also have to push through when we don't feel like training. There's a difference between true exhaustion and making excuses. A good rule of thumb is to train 3-5 times per week, avoiding more than two consecutive rest days.

Consistency is everything. Some days, motivation will be high, and you'll hit your workout hard. Other days, just showing up and checking the box is enough. But as long as you stay disciplined and consistent, you'll keep moving forward—building a strong foundation that will carry you through your career.

Track Your Workouts

We can't know where we're headed unless we understand where we've been. This philosophy is fundamental to training with purpose—progress isn't just about how we feel; it's about measurable, repeatable, and observable results.

Choose a benchmark movement or task and track your performance. For example, if you're performing a 5x5 deadlift, record the weight used for each set. The next time you do the same workout, refer to your previous results and aim to increase the weight by 5 pounds per set. Ideally, by your final set, you'll have set a new personal record.

Fast forward three to six months, and when you retest the movement, your new results will reveal whether your approach was effective. If your performance has improved, your training plan is working. If not, the data provides valuable insights to make adjustments and optimize your progress moving forward.

This isn't just a feeling of getting stronger—it's quantifiable proof of progress in strength, conditioning, and power output. Since the beginning of my fitness journey, I've meticulously recorded nearly every workout. Having this data allows me to validate my progress. On days when things feel tough, or it seems like I'm not advancing, I can look back at the numbers. More often than not, what feels like stagnation is simply a new level of challenge, indicating growth.

Here's my advice: log everything. The good days, the bad days, and even the ones where you're just showing up. Take notes! If you crushed a workout, write down how you felt. If you slept poorly or had a stressful day, note that too. Record how factors like travel, nutrition, and stress impacted your performance. If you set specific goals for the day, like completing all rounds of wall balls unbroken, make a note of it.

Tracking your workouts adds meaning and purpose to your routine. It brings intention to your actions. Just like weighing and measuring your food builds accountability, so does logging your training. For those already dedicated to tracking, you know this to be true. But for those who haven't started, this is your wake-up call! Start tracking, and watch how it transforms your fitness journey.

Stronger On Scene

Equipment Modifications & Substitutions:

The emphasis is on stimulus, not the equipment. If you don't have something a workout calls for, find the next best thing.The goal is to get the same line of action and muscle group as the intended exercise. Barbell, dumbbells and kettlebells can be interchangeable in most workouts.

Below are examples of such modifications

Movement	Substitution
Kettlebells	Dumbbells
Sledge Hammer Strikes	Medicine Ball Slams
Pull Ups	Lat Pulldowns
Chin Ups	Supinated Rows
Hand Over Hand Sled Pull	1-Arm Lat Pulldown
Sled Drag	Ruck Carry
Echo Bike	Any Cardio Machine
Double Unders	2:1 Single Unders
Sandbag over barrier	Over racked barbell

Stronger On Scene

Programming Abbreviations

5/5 : Perform 5 reps on the right side & 5 reps left side

AMRAP: As Many Rounds As Possible

AMREP: As Many Reps As Possible

Alt: Alternate

Ext: Extension

FT: For Time (complete is as quickly as possible)

FR: Front Rack

OH: Overhead

OTM: On The Minute (Every :60)

DB: Dumbbell

DBL: Double

CL/J: Clean & Jerk

KB: Kettlebell

HOH: Hand over hand

Rds: Rounds

(H): Heavy loading; *ability to only do low reps with significant rest*

(M): Moderate loading; *ability to repeatedly be able to do reps*

(L): Light loading; *ability to do many reps without stopping*

Sqt: Squats

ROM: Range of Motion

RFT: Rounds for Time

GHD: Glute Ham Developer

S2OH: Shoulder to overhead (Choice of press, push press, push jerk)

Machine & Distance Conversions

When attempting to convert distances from one modality to another there isn't an exact conversion due to multiple variables. These numbers are also based on Concept 2 ergs, Assault bikes, and the Rogue Echo Bike.

- *For calories and distances not listed use the multipliers provides to get an approximate number.*

Row	Run	Bike Erg	Assault Bike	Echo Bike	Ski Erg
1.25x of Run	.8x of Row	2x of Row	1.25x of Echo	.8x of Assault	1x of Row
250m	200m	500m	15 Calories	12 Calories	250m
500m	400m	1000m	30 Calories	24 Calories	500m
1000m	800m	2000m	60 Calories	48 Calories	1000m
1500m	1200m	3000m	90 Calories	72 Calories	1500m
2000m	1600m	4000m	120 Calories	96 Calories	2000m
5000m	4000m	10,000m	300 Calories	240 Calories	5000m
10,000m	8000m	20,000m	600 Calories	480 Calories	10,000m

Machine & Calorie Conversions

Converting calories between different cardio machines is even less consistent than converting distances. The table below provides general guidance, but it's not exact. When substituting one machine for another while keeping the same rep scheme, consider how long it would take on the given machine. Then, estimate the calories you need to achieve within that timeframe.

Row	Run	Assault Runner	Bike Erg	Assault Bike	Echo Bike	Ski Erg
20 Calories	200m	15 Calories	20 Calories	15 Calories	12 Calories	20 Calories
40 Calories	400m	30 Calories	40 Calories	30 Calories	24 Calories	40 Calories
80 Calories	800m	60 Calories	80 Calories	60 Calories	48 Calories	80 Calories
120 Calories	1200m	90 Calories	120 Calories	90 Calories	72 Calories	120 Calories
160 Calories	1600m	120 Calories	160 Calories	120 Calories	96 Calories	160 Calories
400 Calories	4000m	300 Calories	400 Calories	300 Calories	240 Calories	400 Calories
800 Calories	8000m	600 Calories	800 Calories	600 Calories	480 Calories	800 Calories

Day 1: Full Body Grinder

- 20 Calorie Echo Bike
  10 Sandbag over & jump over barrier *(barrier height 36-42")*
  20 wall balls (30lb/20lb)
  100' Farmer walk (M-H)
- 30 minute AMRAP
  Wear a vest if possible

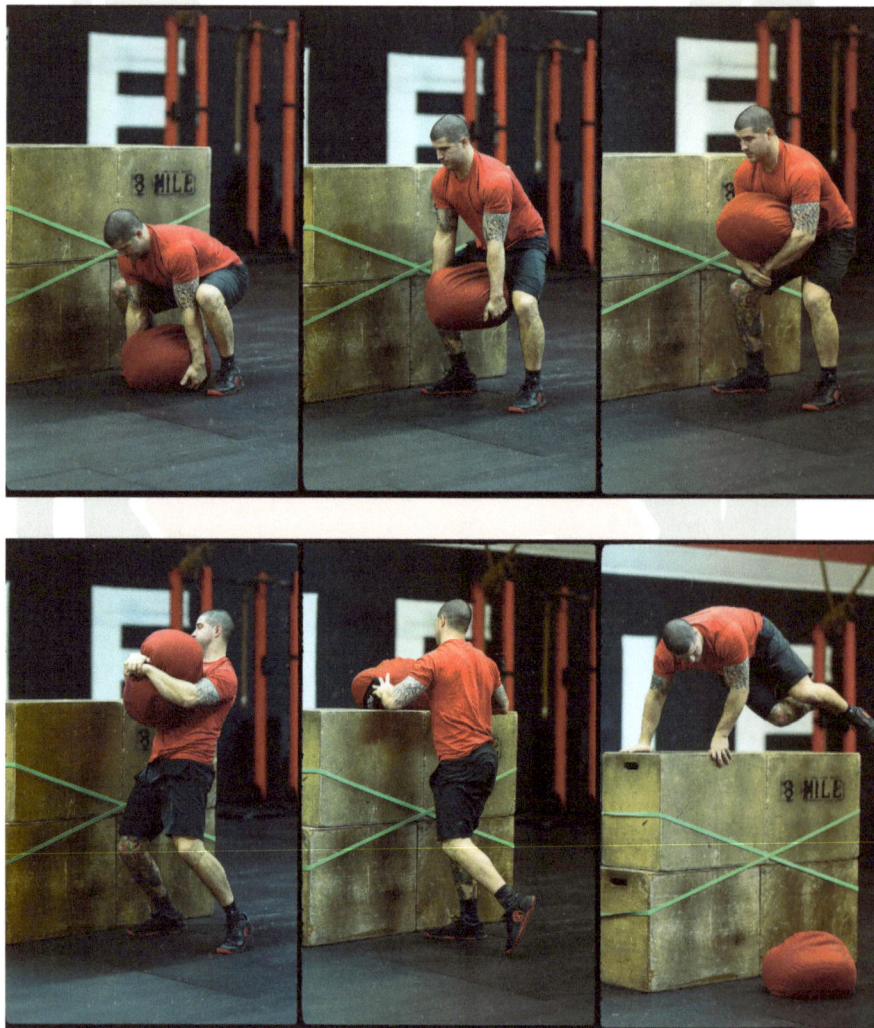

Stronger On Scene

Day 2: Upper Body Lifting

- 10 Bench Press
  7-10 Strict Pull ups
  X5 Sets

- 12 Incline DB Press
  10/10 1-arm DB Row
  X5 sets

- OTM-16minutes-Alt
  10 KB Renegade Rows
  20 Alt KB Press
  10 Chin Ups
  20 1-leg V-Ups

- 20 Alt Bicep Curls
  12 DB Skull Crushers
  X4

- 20 Hammer Curls
  12 Single Arm Tricep Ext
  x3 sets

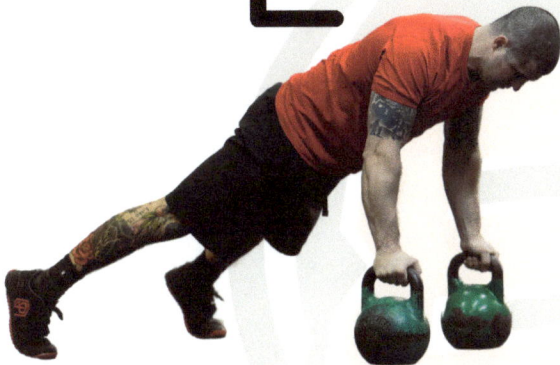

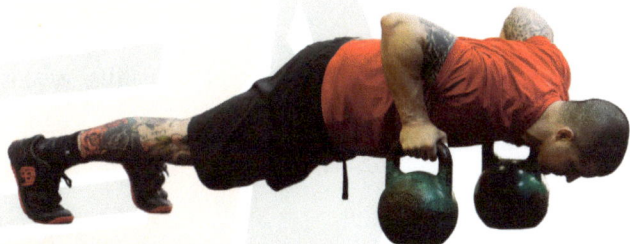

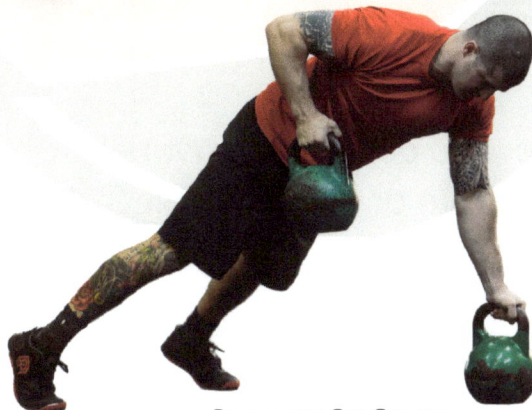

Stronger On Scene

Day 3: Lower Body +Conditioning

- Back Squat: Work up to a heavy single over 20 minutes

- 5/5 Weighted Step ups (H)
- :30 Plank Hold
  - X4 sets

Perform the 3 couplets below without rest between

- 20 Russian KB Swings (M-H)
- 400m Run
  - 3 Rds
- 15 Goblet Squats (M-H)
- 200m Run
  - 3 Rds
- 10 Goblet Squat Clean (M-H)
- 100m Sprints
  - 3 Rds
- -All For Time-

- 10 minutes of Mobility work

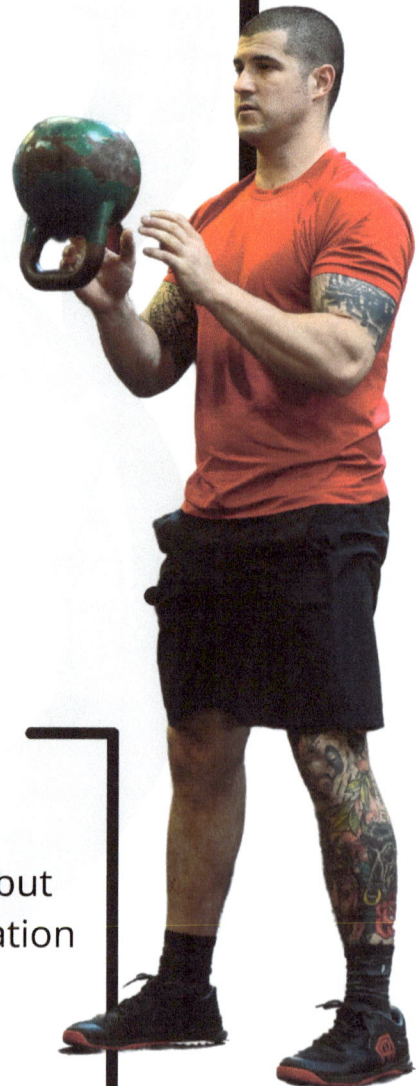

Day 4: Rest

Move to do recovery work but no strain or excessive elevation of the heart rate

Day 5: Full Body Grinder

Partner Training: Partner does 1 full round then switch

- 400m Run/500m Row
  100' DB Bear Crawl (M)
  50' HOH sled pull (M)
  10 Sledge Strikes
  100' Sandbag carry (M-H)
  5 Rds each
- -For Time-

If done solo then change it to a 25 minute AMRAP

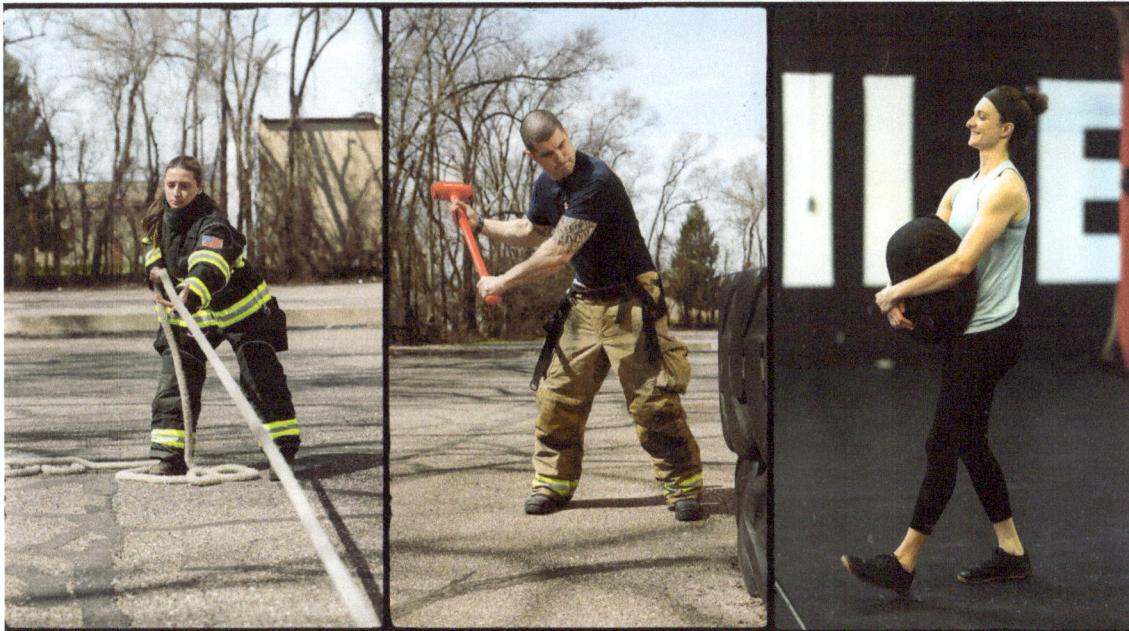

Day 6: Lower Body+Conditioning

- Front Squat: Work up to a heavy single over 20 minute

- 7/7 Bulgarian split squats
  10 OH KB Sit ups
  X4
- 21's Goblet Squats
  - 7 Reps Top ½ ROM
  - 7 Reps Bottom ½ ROM
  - 7 Reps Full ROM
    - that equals one round

Perform 3 total rounds

- 3 minute Stair Stepper
  10/10 KB/DB SN (M)
  4 Rounds

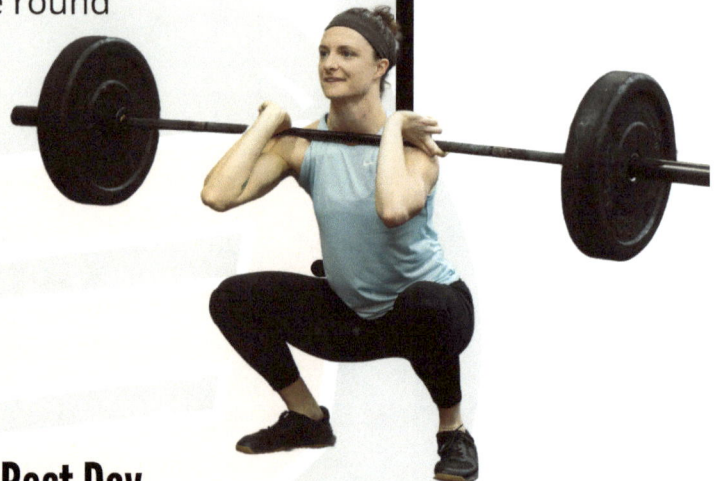

Day 7: Rest Day

Play a sport, get 10k steps in, but no traditional weight training or cardio

Day 8: Upper Body Lifting

- 10-8-6
  Deficit Push Ups
  Strict Pull Ups

Then

- 16 Sledge strikes
  Repeat all of the above for 3 cycles

- 10 Incline DB Curls
  15 DB OH Tricep Ext
  X3

- 12 Hammer Curls
  12 Tate Press
  x4

- 1x100 Banded Pull Aparts

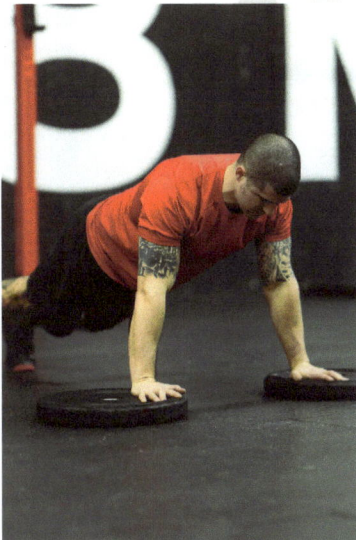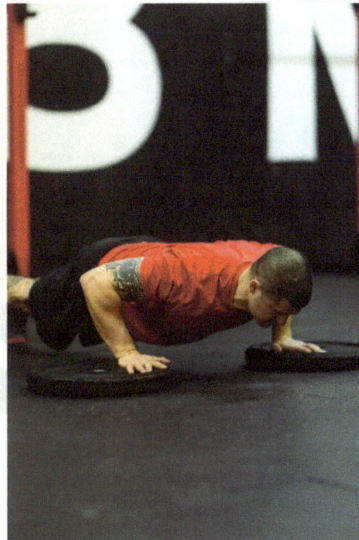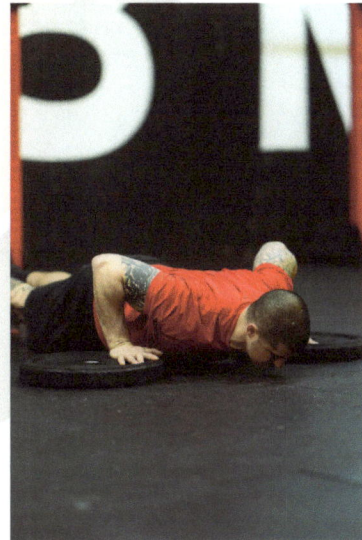

Day 9: Lower Body Lifting

- Deadlift: Work up to a heavy single over 20 minutes

- 10 Russian KB swings (H)
  10 Goblet Squats (H)
  10 GHD Sit ups or 20 V-ups
  X5 sets

- 50' Walking Weighted Lunge (M-H)
  20 KB/DB Pull Throughs (M)
  X4 sets

- 10 Cossack Squats
  10 Calf Raises
  X4 -Not for intensity

- 4 Min Sled Drag Forward (L-M)
- 4 Min Sled Drag Backwards

- :10 Echo Bike Sprint
  :20 Echo Bike Slow
  8 Rds

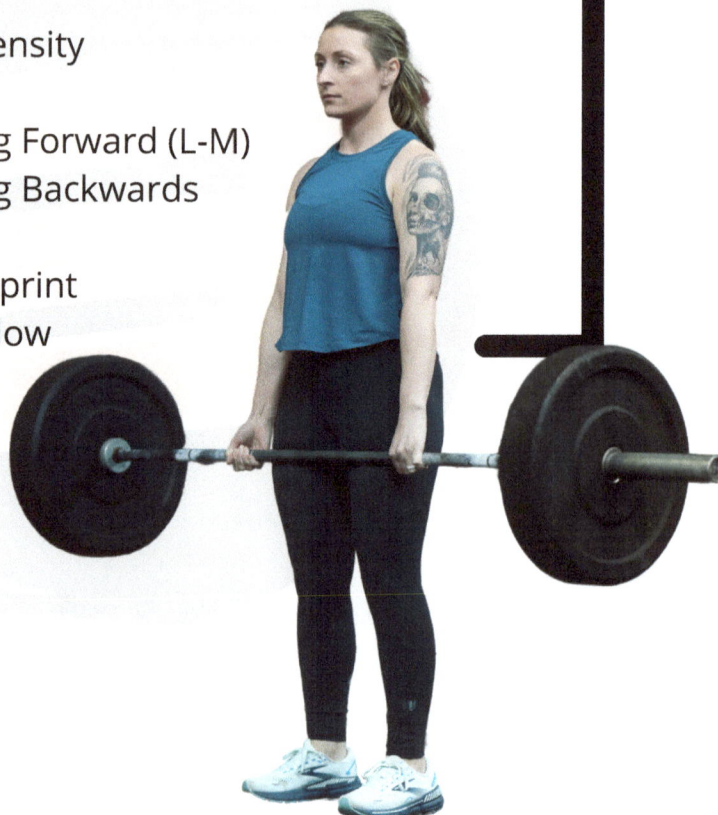

Stronger On Scene

Day 10: Conditioning

- 400m Run
  500m Row
  100m Farmer Carry (M)
25 minute AMRAP

10 minute Mobility Work

Day 11: Rest

Play a sport, get 10k steps in, but no traditional weight training or cardio

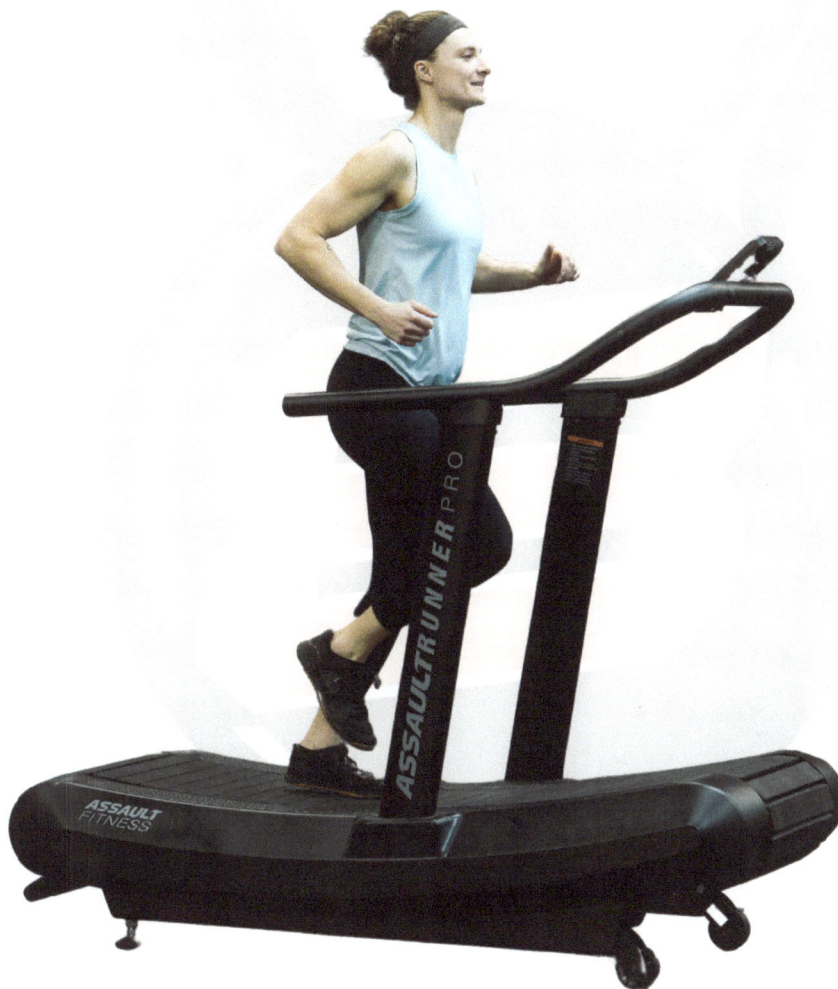

Stronger On Scene

Day 12: Upper Body Grinder

- 8 Alt Gorilla Rows
  4 FR Kneeling to standing
  8 S2OH
  4 Shuttle runs

- 10 Alt Gorilla Rows
  5 FR Kneeling to standing
  10 S2OH
  5 Shuttle runs

- 12 Alt Gorilla Rows
  6 FR Kneeling to standing
  12 S2OH
  6 Shuttle runs
Continue this rep progression for 12 minutes

  3 minute Rest then

- :20 Work :20 Rest x10
  Ski Erg or Air Bike

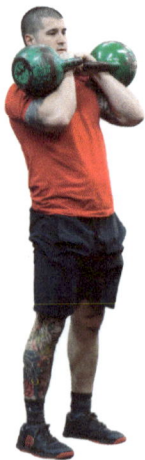

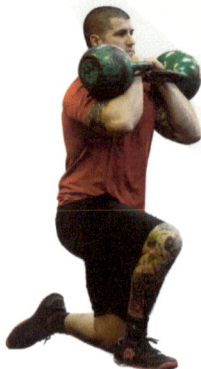

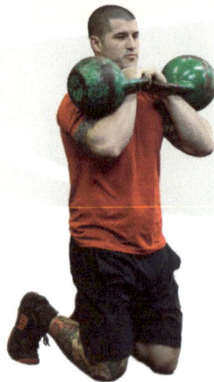

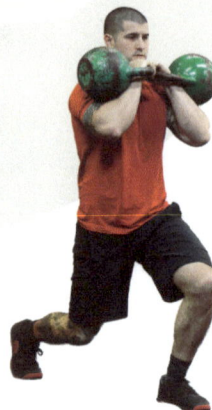

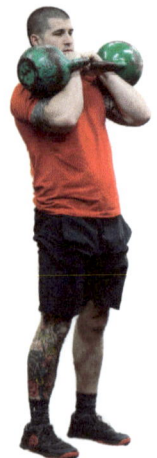

Stronger On Scene

Day 13: Lower Body Lifting

- 5x5 Back Squat at 70-85% of 1RM

- 4x 7/7 Back Rack Reverse Lunge (M)

- 4x10 Explosive KB Deadlift (M-H)

- OTM-5 minute
  7 Goblet Cyclist Squats (H)

- Pick 1 : Stair stepper: 15 minute of intervals
      2 Mile Run
      3k Row

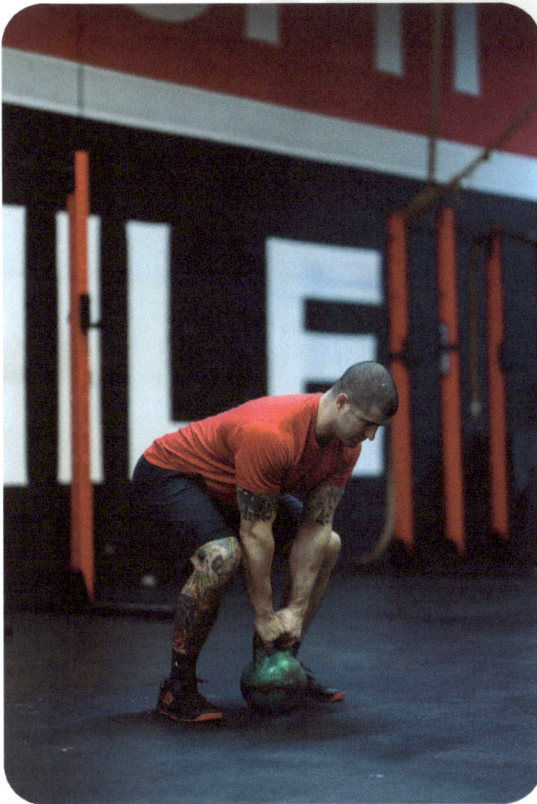

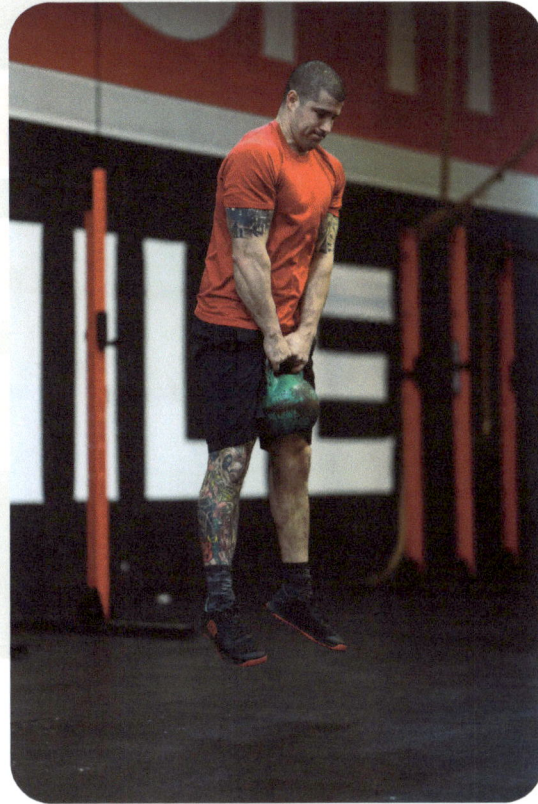

Stronger On Scene

Day 14: Rest

Go get a massage, do yoga, loosen the body up without elevating the heart rate

Day 15: Upper Body Grinder

- 500m Row(+250m each round)
  20 Box Step ups (+10 each round)
  50' (1) KB/DB Bear crawl (+ 50' each round)
  50' DBL FR walking lunge(+50' each round
  20 gorilla rows (+10 each round)
  30 minute AMRAP
- **with a vest if possible**

- 10 minute Mobility Work

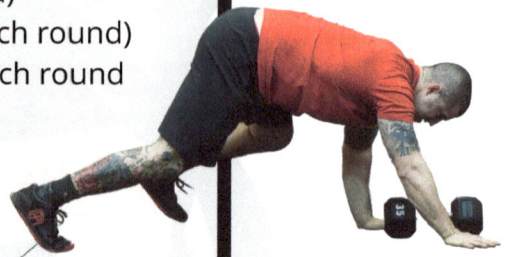

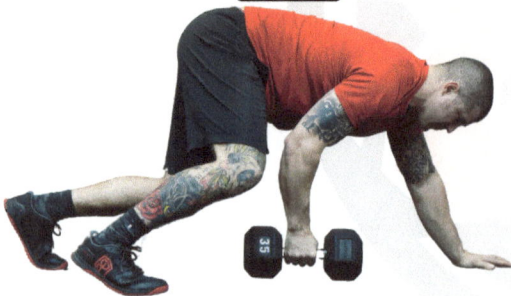

Day 16: Conditioning+Full Body

- 1minute Stations for Max Effort
  Air Bike
  Sledge Strikes
  Double Unders/Jump rope
  Burpees
  V-Ups
  Rest 1 minute
  4 Rounds

Stronger On Scene

Effort Is a Choice

Most jobs in emergency services and the military require a physical fitness standard before hiring. It's a baseline—a minimum threshold you must meet to even be considered. And yet, with staffing shortages across the country, some agencies are lowering or even removing that requirement.

I've seen countless people train relentlessly to meet that standard, pushing themselves to earn their place. But here's the reality: that was just the beginning. Meeting the entry-level requirement took effort, but maintaining and exceeding that standard takes even more.

Congratulations—you got the job! You're now a firefighter, police officer, or military professional. But now the real work begins. Too many men and women grow complacent once they're in. The truth is, our jobs don't demand peak performance every single day—but when they do, lives are on the line. And even when we're not at 100%, we still need to operate at 80-85% efficiency on a regular basis.

I don't know about you, but I have a wife and kids to go home to. My partner has a daughter who dreams of being walked down the aisle one day. When the moment comes, I need to be ready—no excuses, no second chances.

Effort is a choice. Every day, you decide whether to put in the work. Whether to train with intention. Whether to stay fit, eat right, and hold yourself accountable. You made a commitment to serve others—your community, your team, and your loved ones. That commitment doesn't end when you clock out.

Readiness isn't a one-time achievement—it's a responsibility. Choose to be ready. Choose to put in the effort.

Day 17: Full Body Conditioning

- OTM-30 minute-Alt
  15 Wall Balls
  15-25 Push Ups
  10-15 DL (L-M)
  10-15 Pull Ups
  12-15 Calorie Row

Day 18: Rest

- Stay active but recover

Day 19: Upper Body+Conditioning

- 2 minute AMRAP
  10 Burpees
  7 DBL KB Clean (M)
  7 DBL KB Push Press
  7 DBL KB CL/J

1 minute Rest

- 2 minute AMRAP
  50' HOH Sled pull (M)
  50' Sled push
  50' HOH Sled pull
  50' Sled push

1 minute Rest

4 Cycles of everything Above

- 8 Reps of Each: *Unbroken Rounds*
  Upright rows
  Bicep Curls
  Strict Press
  Hang Power CL/J
  Bent over Rows
  X3 Rounds- rest as needed

Stronger On Scene

Day 20: Lower Body Lifting

- 5x5 Front Squat at 70-85% of 1RM

- 12 DB Dimmel DL
  10 OH KB Sit ups
  X5 Sets

- 100' Weighted Lunges (M)
  15 Goblet Squats
  x4 Sets

- OTM-14 minute- Alt
  100' Sled push (H)
  100' 1-arm Farmer Carry (H)

- Pick 1 : 10 minute Stair stepper Level 7+*vest*
          1 Mile Run Time Trial
          2k Row

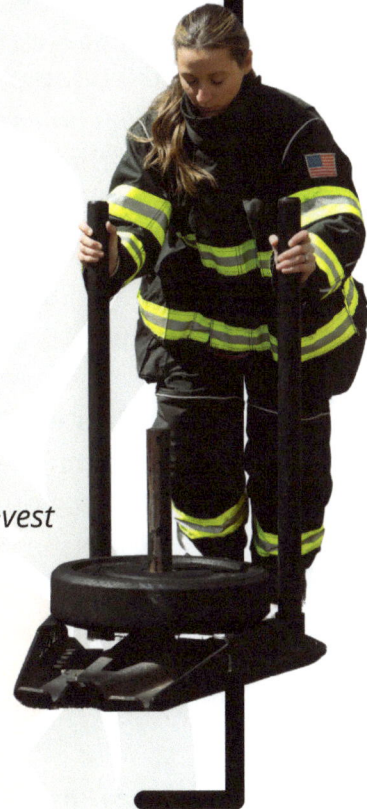

Day 21: Rest

- Stay active but recover

Day 22: Conditioning+Full Body

- 30 Cal Bike
  10 Burpees over sandbag
  10 Sandbag Squats (M)
  20 Sit ups
  5RFT

Day 23: Conditioning+Upper Body Lifting

- 3:00 AMRAP /3:00 Rest
  x5 Intervals
  10-15 Cal Bike
  30 Double Unders /60 Single Unders
  With time remaining: Max Rep Power Clean & Jerks
  (barbell/DB/KB/Plate G2OH)

- 8 DB Incline Bench
  7-10 Pull ups
  X6 Sets

- 12 Lateral DB Raise
  12 Front DB Raise
  15 Face pulls (Cable or Band)
  X3 sets

- 10 Incline DB Curls
  15 DB OH Tricep Ext
  X3

- 12 Hammer Curls
  12 Tate Press
  x4

- 1x100 Banded Pull aparts

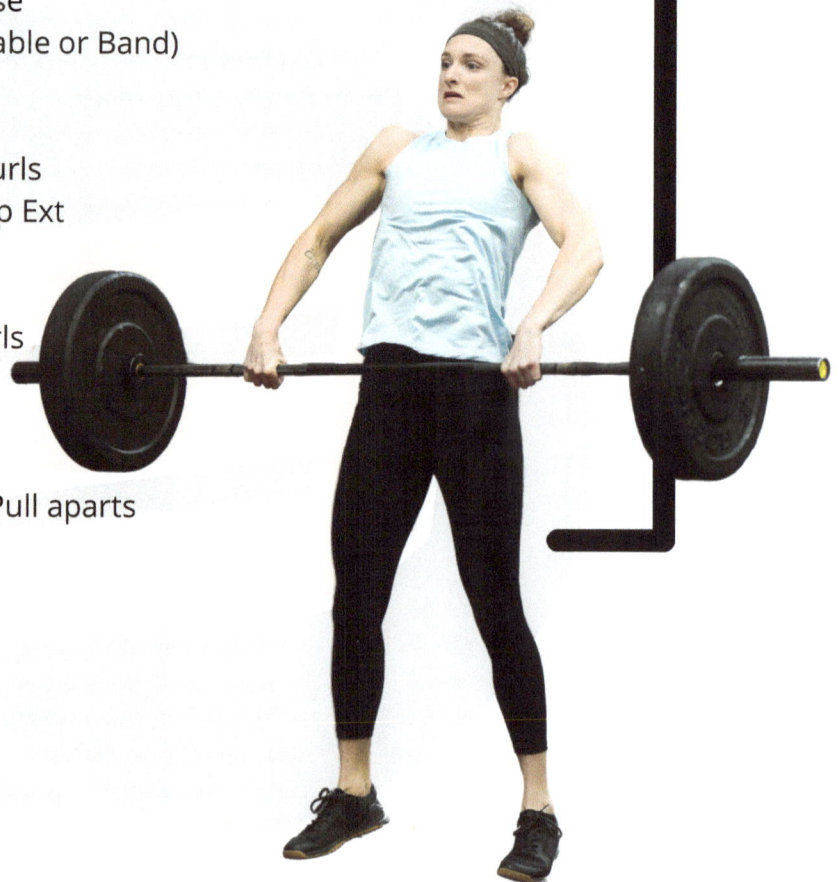

Stronger On Scene

Day 24: Lower Body Lifting

- 5x5 Deadlift at 70-85% of 1RM

- 4x 6/6 BR Reverse Lunge

- OTM-5 minute
  7 DBL KB FSQ

- 8 Back Ext
  :30 L-Sit Hold
  x4 sets

- 12 Weighted V-Ups
  10 Hip Thrusts (H)
  X4 Set

- Pick 1 :
  - Stair stepper + Vest
    - :45 90 s/m
    - :45 42 s/m
      x6
  - 2 Mile Run
  - 200m Sprint 100m Walk x7

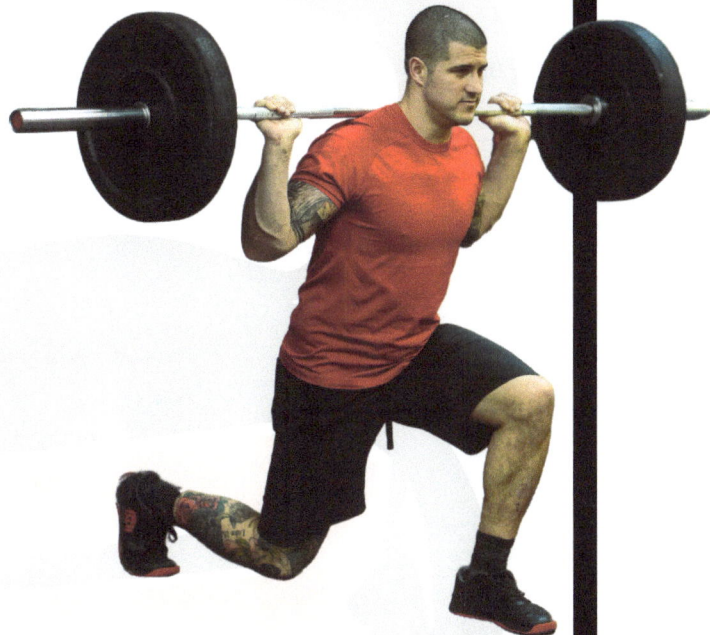

Day 25: Rest

- Stay active but recover

Stronger On Scene

Day 26: Full Body Grinder

- 10 Burpee Over Box
  50' Sled push
  50' sled drag
  :60 sandbag Bear Hug Hold
  2 minute rest
  X5 Rounds

Burpee over chest height barrier to increase difficulty

Day 27: Full Body Grinder

- 10 Thrusters (M- H)
  20 Pull ups
  30 Push Ups
  40 Sit Ups
  50 ASQ
  3 minute Rest
4 Rounds For Time

Vest optional

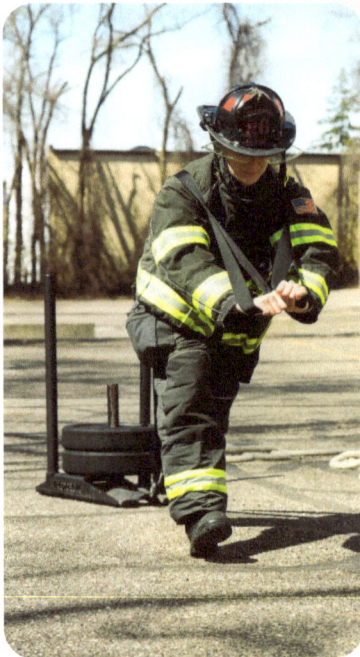

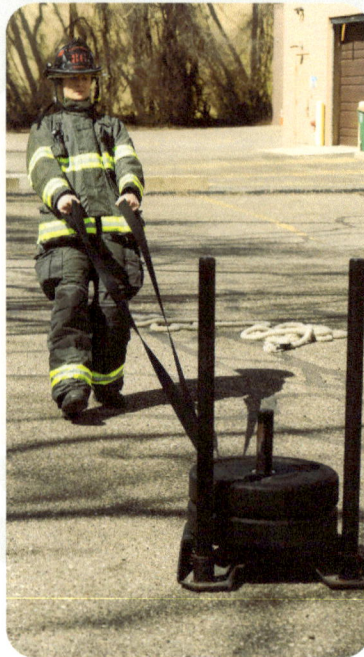

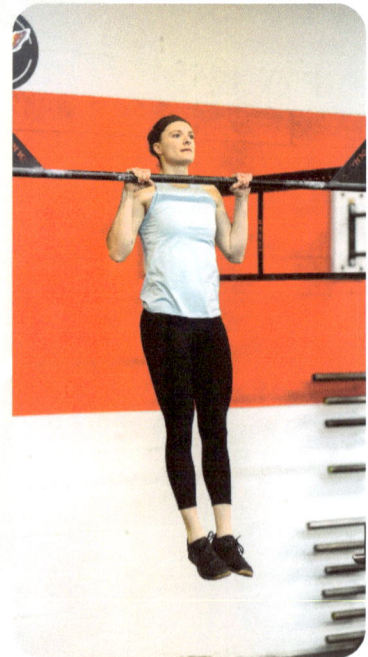

Stronger On Scene

Day 28: Rest

- Rest up for a retest workout the following day

- Refer to day 1 results to have a training goal to beat

Day 29: Full Body Grinder

- 20 Calorie Echo Bike
  10 Sandbag over & jump over barrier
  (barrier height 36-42")
  20 wall balls (30lb/20lb)
  100' Farmer walk
  30 minute AMRAP

Use vest if you used it on day 1, and same loading as day 1

- 4 Min Sled Drag Forward
- 4 Min Sled Drag Backwards

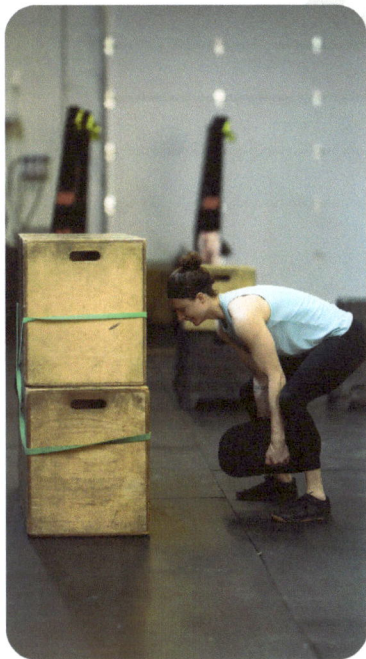

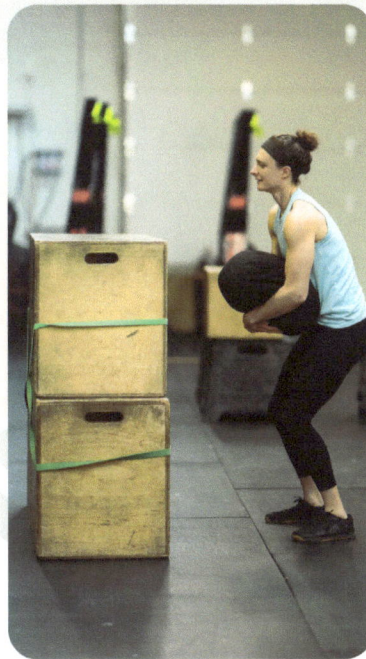

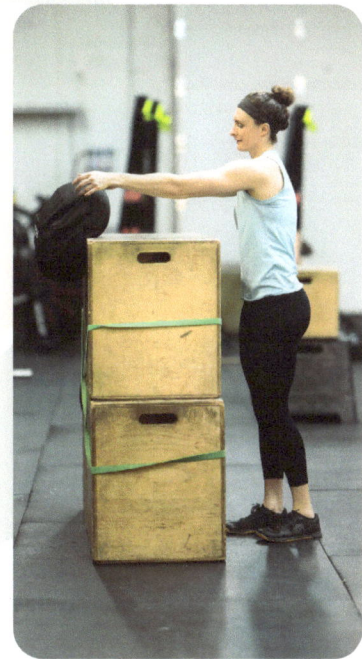

Day 30: Upper Body Lifting

- 7-10 DB Bench Press (H)
  Right into max rep incline push ups
  :90 Rest
  X4 sets

- 3 Weighted Pull ups
  10 Weighted Dips
  x7 Sets

- 8 Reps of Each: *Unbroken Rounds*
  Upright rows
  Bicep Curls
  Strict Press
  Hang Power CL/J
  Bent over Rows
  X3 Rounds- *rest as needed*

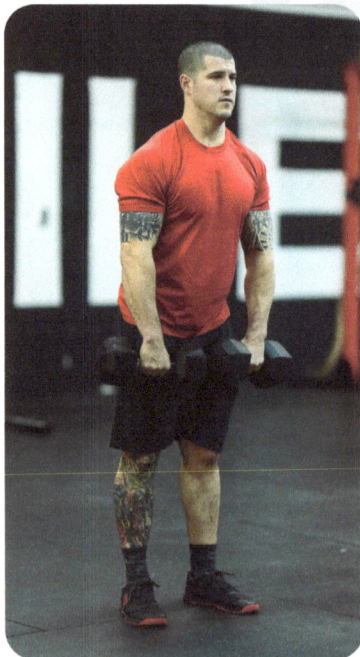

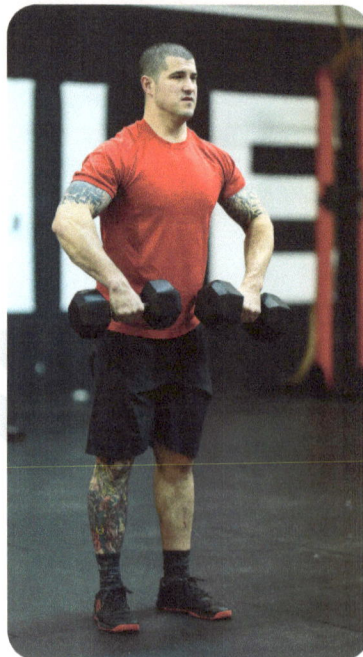

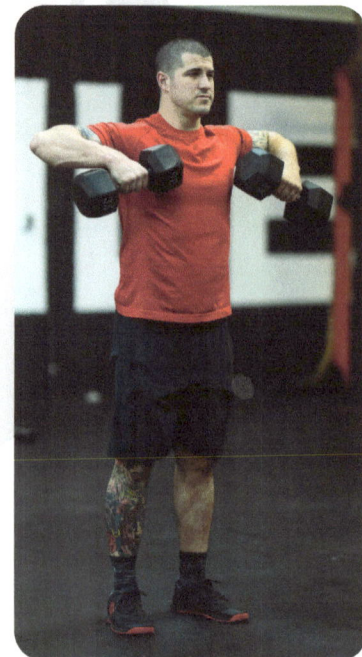

Stronger On Scene

Day 31: Conditioning + Lower Body Lifting

- 5x3 FSQ at 85-95% of 1RM

- 400m Run
  15 Goblet Squats (M-H) KB/DB
  20 Russian KB Swings (M)
  100m Farmer's Carry (heavy)
  4 Rounds for Time

- 4x 6/6 BR Reverse Lunge

- 3x15 Hanging Knee Raises

- 3x30 Weighted Side Bends
  (each side)

- 4 Min Sled Drag Forward
- 4 Min Sled Drag Backwards

Day 32: Rest

Pick 1:
- Find a Yoga Class to attend!
- Go hike
- Walk 15k steps

Day 33: Lower Body Lifting

- Back Squat: Work up to a heavy 3-rep max over 20 minute

- 4x6 Tempo Front Squat (3-1-1)

- 4x10 Romanian Deadlifts (M-H)

- 3x12 Box Step-Ups (weighted)

- OTM-5minute
  10-12 Goblet Cyclist Squats

Stronger On Scene

Day 34: Rest

Pick 1:
- Find a Yoga Class to attend!
- Go hike
- Walk 15k steps

Day 35: Full Body + Grinder

- 15 Calorie Row
  10 Sandbag Cleans (M-H)
  50' DB Bear Crawl (M)
  50' DBL DB FR Walking Lunge (M)
  10 Burpee box jump overs (30"/24")
  100' Farmers Carry (H)
  5RFT

- 3x30 Russian Twists (weighted)
- 3x20 Hanging Knee Raises
- 3x :20 L-Sit Hold

Are You Tracking Your Workouts?

Tracking your training sessions—recording weights, reps, times, and progressions—is key to seeing improvement. Without it, how will you know if you're getting stronger or faster?

A training log keeps you accountable, highlights progress, and helps set clear goals to keep pushing forward.

Day 36: Conditioning + Upper Body Lifting

- 4 minute AMRAP
100m Run
5 KB Renegade Row
5 KB CLs
5 KB Push Jerks
5 KB CL/J

1 minute Rest

- 4min AMRAP
100m Run
50' HOH Sled Pull
50' Sled push

1 minute Rest

4 Cycles of everything Above

- 8x8 Barbell bent over Rows
- 3x12 Lat pulldowns
- 3x15 Cable face pulls
- 3x10 Hammer curls

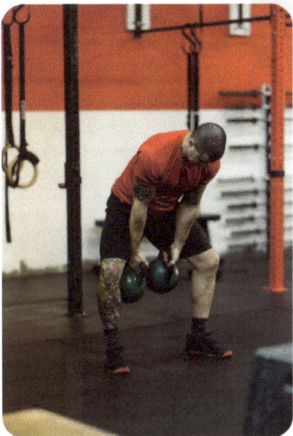

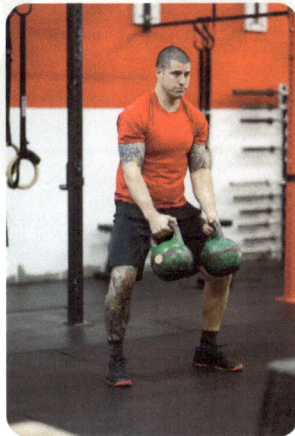

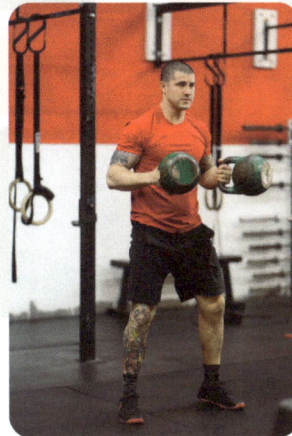

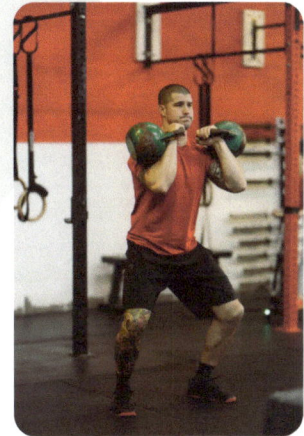

Stronger On Scene

Day 37: Lower Body Lifting+Conditioning

- FSQ: Work up to a heavy 1-rep max over 20 minute

- 4x6/6 Bulgarian Split Squats

- 4x8 Explosive KB DLs (H)

- OTM-12 minute-Alt
  100' sled push (H)
  100' 1-arm Farmer Carry (H)

- :20 **Sprint** :40 Moderate to low intensity x12 Intervals
  - Your choice of method

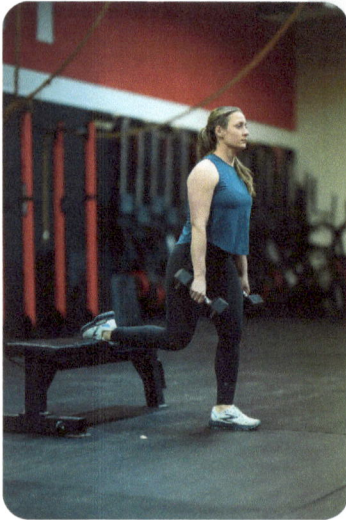

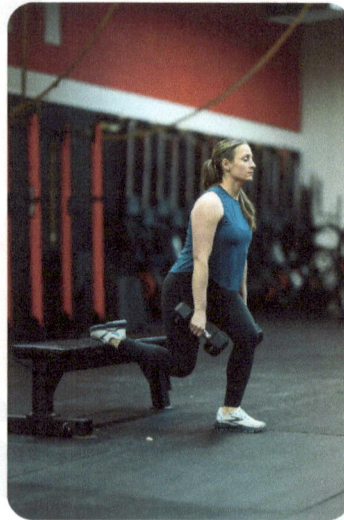

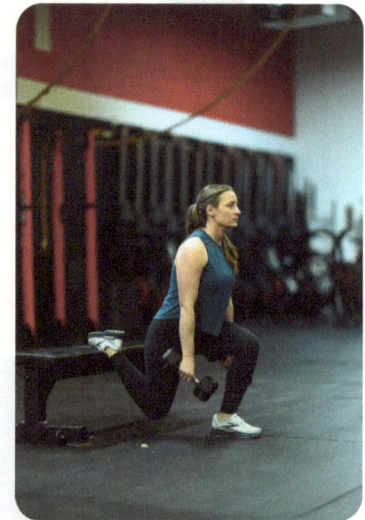

Day 38: Rest

Pick 1:
- Find a Yoga Class to attend!
- Go hike
- Walk 15k steps

Day 39: Conditioning+Full Body

- OTM-20 minute- Alt
  12 Russian KB Swings (H)
  :20 L-Sit Hold

- 30 Calorie bike
  20 Sledge Strike/Med Ball Slams
  10 BR Lunges (M)
  4RFT

- 3x10 Hanging Toes 2 bar
- 3x20 Med ball Russian twists

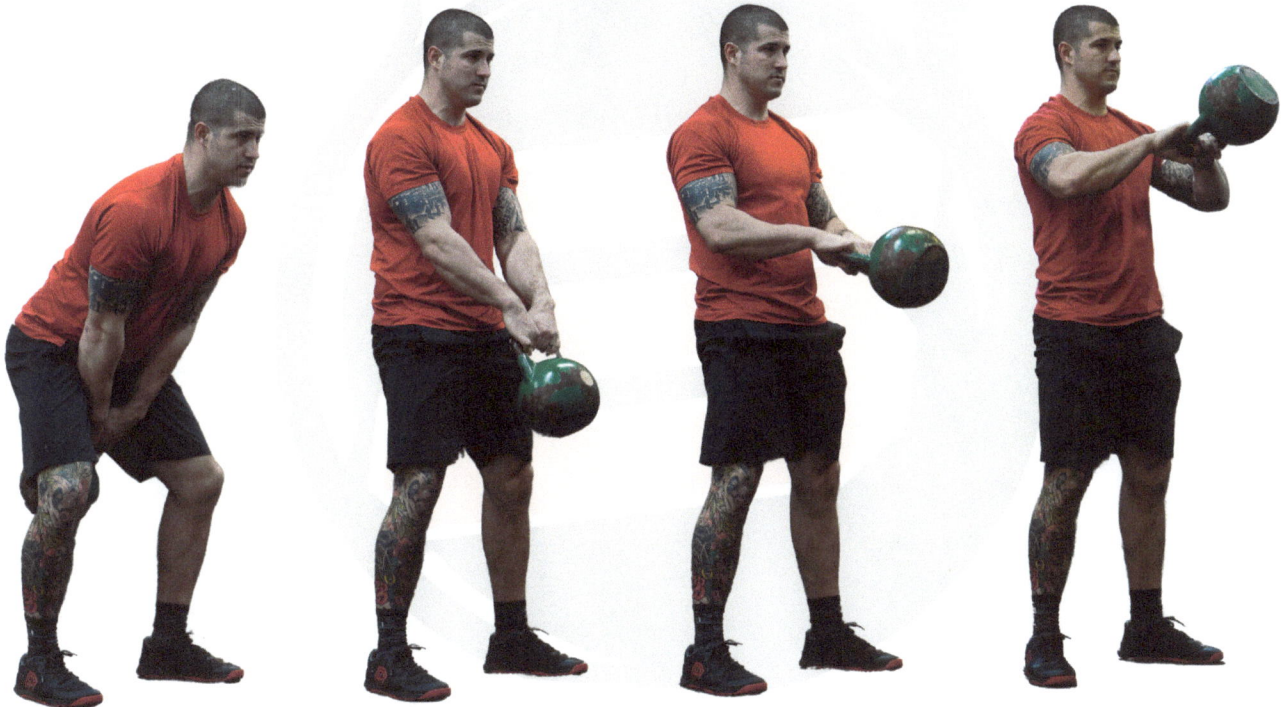

Day 40:Upper Body Grinder

- 500m Row/400m Run
  20 Strict Press (M)
  20 Bent Over Rows (M)
  20 Burpees
  :90 Rest
- Repeat; reducing reps by 5.
  Rd 2: Reps of 15, Rd 3 Reps of 10

- 8 Incline DB Bench Press
  7-10 strict pull ups
  X5 sets

- 4x8 Seated DB OH Press
- 4x12 DB Front & Lateral Raises
- 3x15 Cable/Band Facepulls
- 1x100 Banded pull aparts

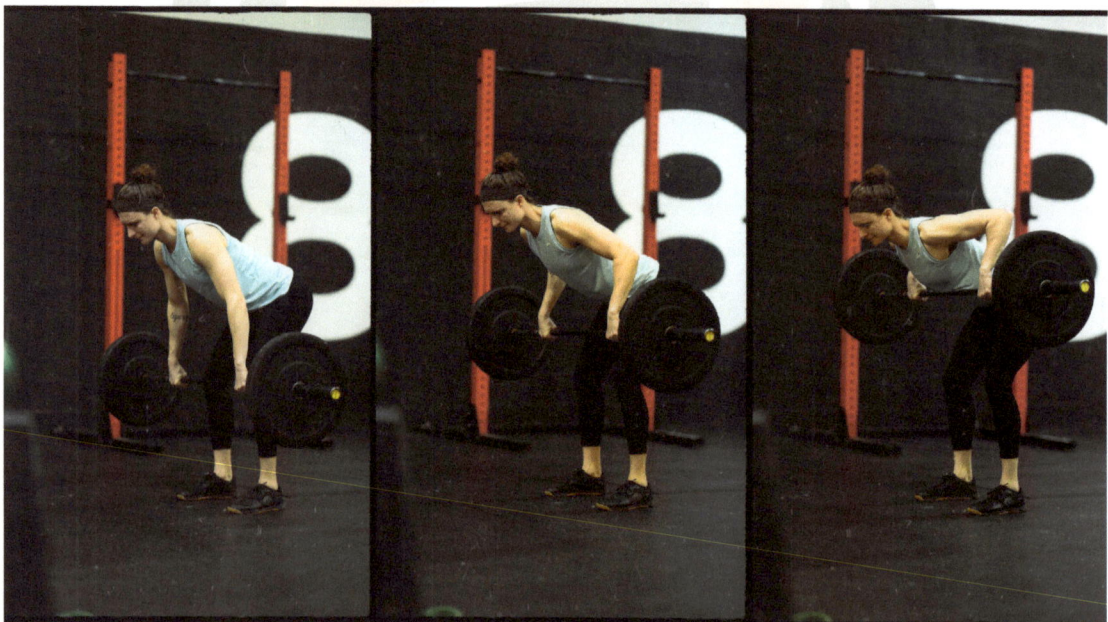

Stronger On Scene

Day 41: Lower Body Lifting

- Back Squat: 7x1 a work up to a heavy single

- 4x10/10 Back Rack Reverse Lunge

- 3x12 DB Dimmel DL

- OTM-5 minute
  7 DBL KB FSQ

- 3x10 Hip thrusts (H)

- 4 Min Sled Drag Forward
  4 Min Sled Drag Backwards

Pick 1: :45 Fast :90 Moderate x8 Rds
Stair Stepper/ Run/ Row/ Bike

Day 42: Rest Day

Making progress? GREAT
- If not, where can we be better?
  - Sleep?
  - Nutrition?
  - Mobility?
  - Reduce stimulants?
  - Intensity?
  - Consistency?

Day 43: Conditioning+Upper Body

- E3M x6
  200' Sled Push (L-M)
  15-20 Push ups
  7-10 Power Clean (Barbell, DB, KB)
  200' Farmer Walk

- 8 Reps of Each: *Unbroken Rounds*
  Upright rows
  Bicep Curls
  Strict Press
  Hang Power CL/J
  Bent over Rows
  X3 Rounds- rest as needed

Day 44: Lower Body Lifting

- Deadlift: Work up to a heavy 3-rep max over 20 minute

- 4x6/6 Back Rack Reverse Lunge

- 4x10 Front squats

- 3x12 Cossack Squats (controlled, not for speed)

- OTM-10 minute:
  7 Goblet Cyclist Squats
  10 Weighted Calf Raises

- 3x20 Weighted Sit-ups
- 3x:30 L-Sit Hold

- :20 **Sprint** :40 Moderate to low intensity x12 Intervals *Your choice of method*

Day:45 Test Day

You've been grinding, pushing through the pain, and showing up when it counts. But this isn't just about training—it's about the job. The mission. The calling to be the one who steps up when others are in need.

Now it's time to prove it. Time to put your strength, endurance, and willpower to the test. No excuses. No hesitation. Just action.

Go take your industry's candidate physical test.
 CPAT – MCOLES – PFT
Step up. Own it. Earn it.

Don't have all the equipment? Simulate or substitute as you need and do a couple rounds but ensuring to hit the high spots of the test.

Too Easy? Do multiple rounds. Create a new test for you.

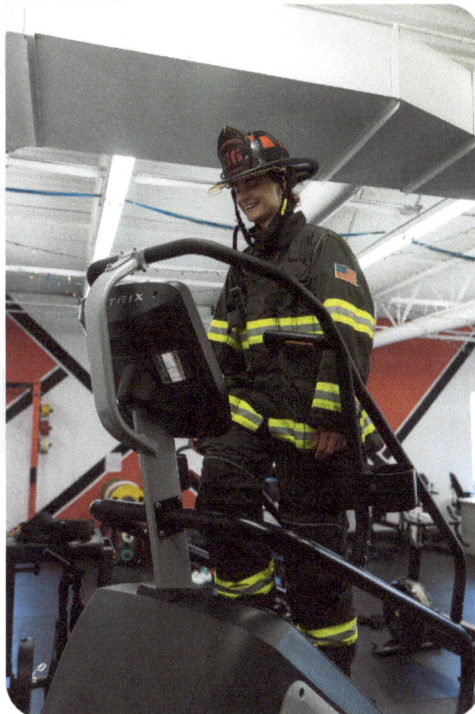

Stronger On Scene

MCOLES: Michigan Commission on Laws Enforcement Standards

Age and Gender Dependent*

Event 1: Max Vertical Jump in 3 attempts
Event 2: Max Sit Ups in :60
Event 3: Max Push Ups in :60
Event 4: Max Half Mile Shuttle Run

Male Pre-Enrollment Physical Fitness Test Score – Minimum Requirements

Age Group	Vertical Jump	Sit-Ups	Push-Ups	½ -Mile Shuttle Run
18-29	17.5	32	30	4:29.6
30-39	16.0	30	30	4:38.2
40+	15.0	30	28	4:54.7

Male Exit Physical Fitness Test– Minimum Requirements

Age Group	Vertical Jump	Sit-Ups	Push-Ups	½ -Mile Shuttle Run
18-29	19.0	36	37	4:11.8
30-39	17.5	34	37	4:18.2
40+	16.5	34	35	4:27.8

Female Pre-Enrollment Physical Fitness Test– Minimum Requirements

Age Group	Vertical Jump	Sit-Ups	Push-Ups	½ -Mile Shuttle Run
18-29	11.0	28	7	5:35.4
30-39	9.0	19	7	5:59.1
40+	8.0	18	7	6:13.3

Female Exit Physical Fitness Test– Minimum Requirements

Age Group	Vertical Jump	Sit-Ups	Push-Ups	½ -Mile Shuttle Run
18-29	12.0	32	12	5:02.6
30-39	10.0	23	12	5:19.0
40+	9.0	20	11	5:25.5

Stronger On Scene

CPAT: Candidate Physical Agility Test

8 station course to be completed with a max allotted time of 10 minutes and 20 seconds. Course to be completed with 50lb weight vest

- 3 minutes 20 seconds Stair Stepper with 75lb vest
- Hose Drag
- Equipment Carry
- Ladder Raise & Extension
- Forcible Entry
- Maze Search
- Victim Drag
- Ceiling Breach & Pull

Common Stations of Failed Tests:

1. Stair Stepper
2. Forcible Entry
3. Victim Drag

ACFT: Army Combat Fitness Test

Scoring is different based on gender and age.

- 3 Rep Max Deadlift (Trap Bar)

- Standing Power Throw (10 lbs Medicine Ball)

- Hand Release Push Ups (Reps in 2 Minutes)

- Sprint-Drag-Carry (40 lb KB Carry+90 lb sled)

- Plank (Max Time)

- Two Mile Run

Now What?

You did it. You committed to a program, took ownership of your fitness, and became a stronger member of your team because of it. But you might be asking yourself, "Now what?"

Use this as a launching point to keep building your foundation in fitness and movement. You can repeat this program, aiming to complete it heavier or faster than before. You can tweak and adapt it as you continue training. I encourage you to turn these past 45 days into another 90—until fitness becomes a lifelong priority.

Life won't slow down. You'll navigate relationships, maybe have kids, take on new responsibilities, and get older. Through it all, fitness must remain a priority. By starting now, you're building a foundation that your career—and your future—will stand on. You don't need to be at peak physical fitness every day, but as long as you maintain a solid base, you'll always be ready when the call comes.

Readiness isn't a one-time achievement—it's a responsibility. Choose to be ready. Choose to put in the effort.

Movement Appendix

Squat Variations

Back Squat

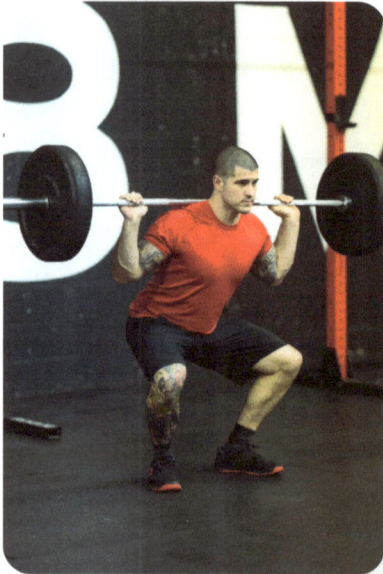

Front Squat

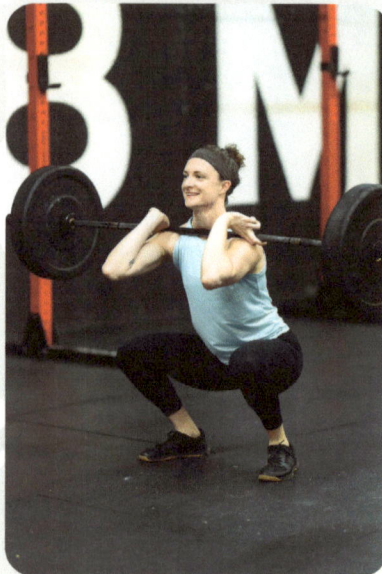

Goblet Squat

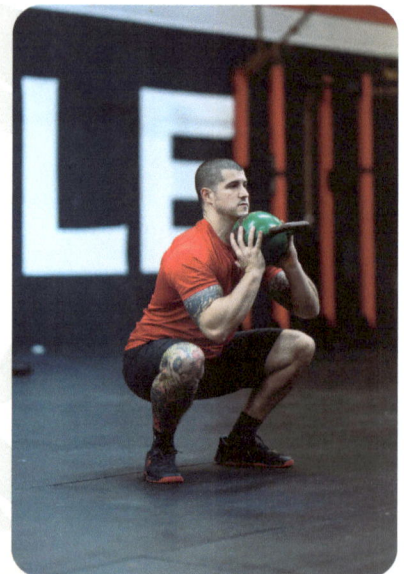

Double Kettlebell Front Squat

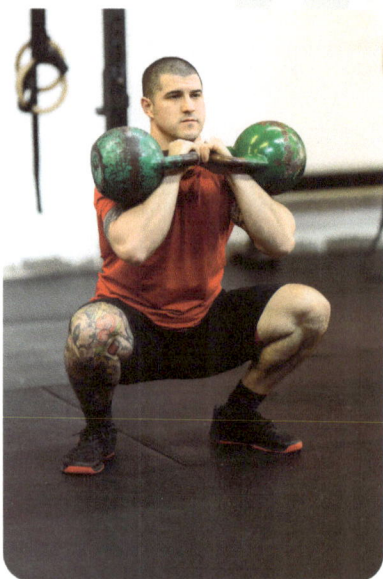

Single Kettlebell Squat

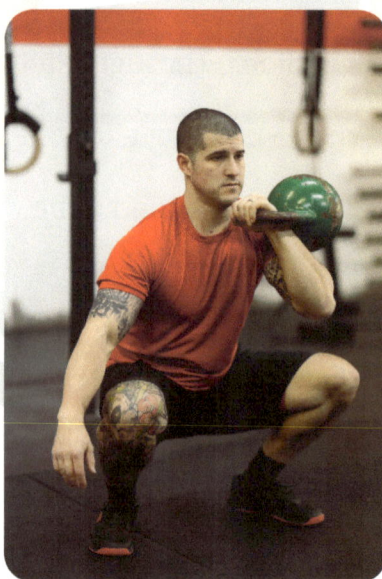

Goblet Cyclist Squat

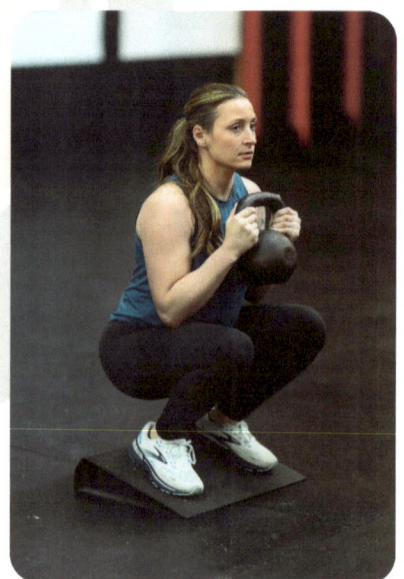

Movement Appendix

Squat Variations

Wall Balls

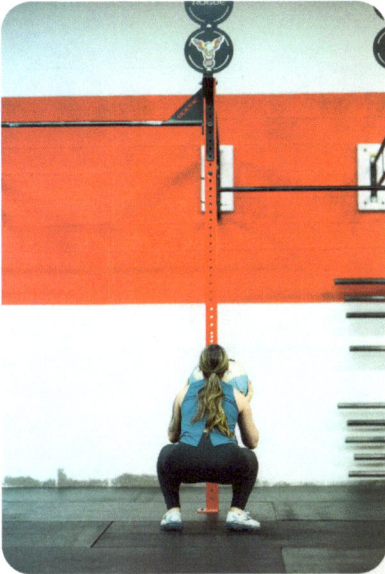 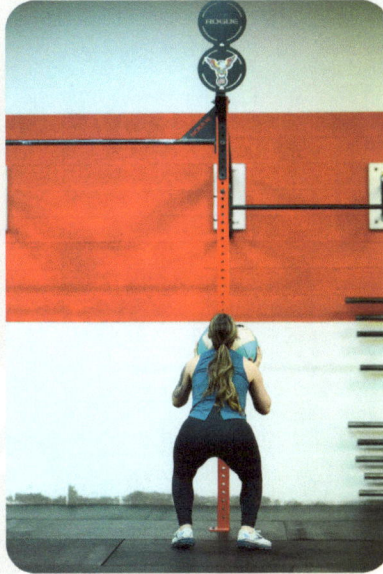 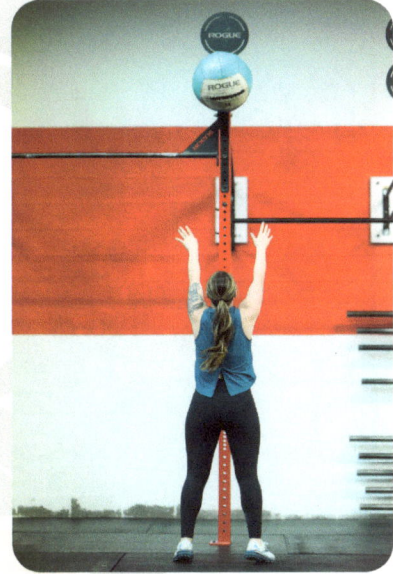

Thrusters

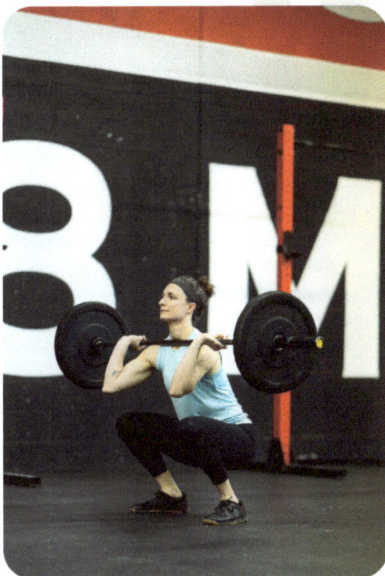 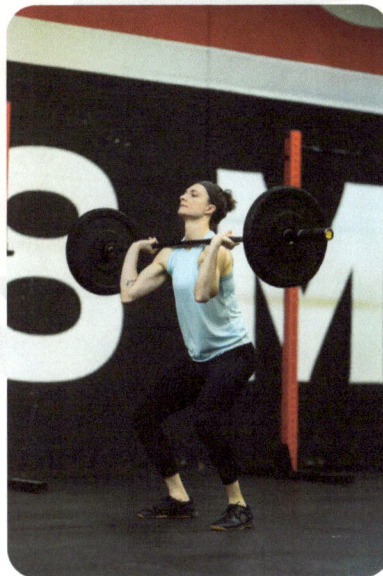 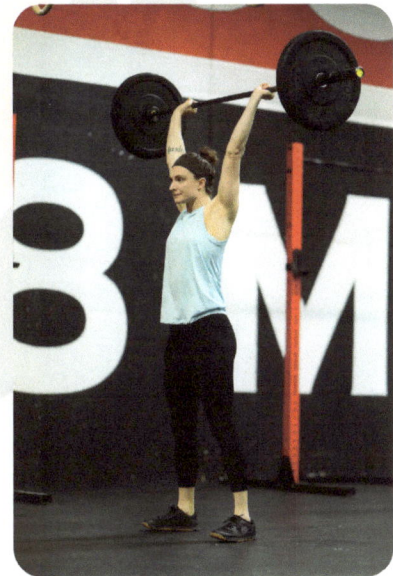

Stronger On Scene

Movement Appendix

Squat Variations

Kettlebell Swing to Goblet Squat

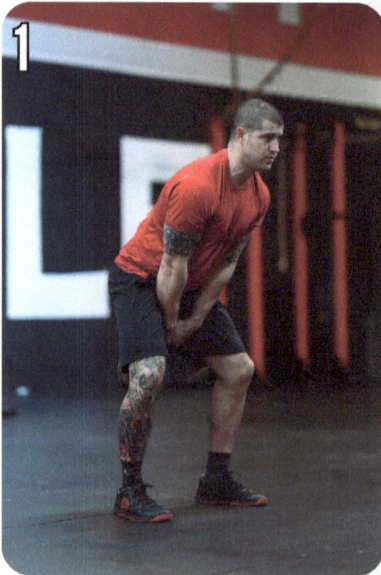

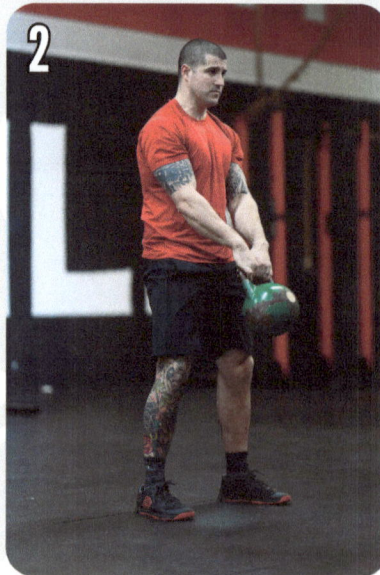

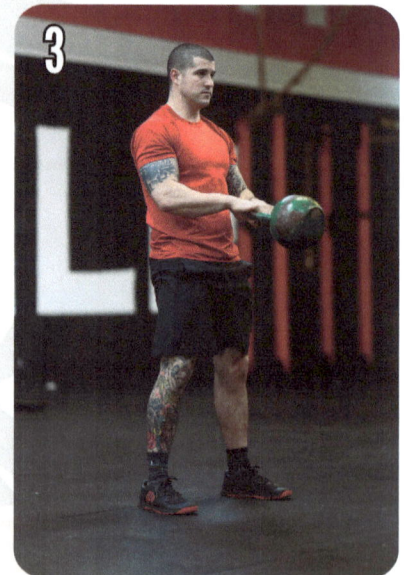

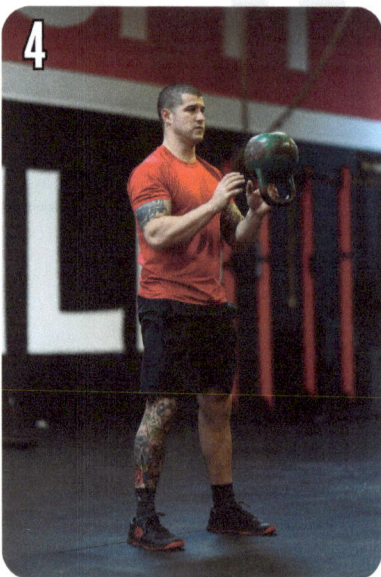

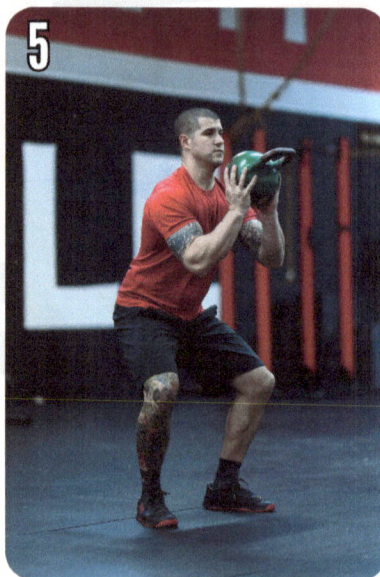

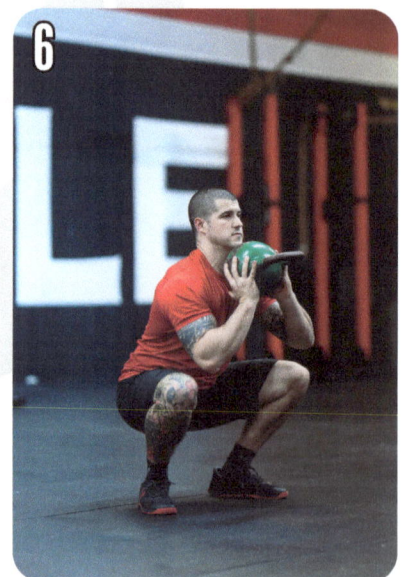

Stronger On Scene

Movement Appendix
Squat Variations

Bulgarian Split Squats

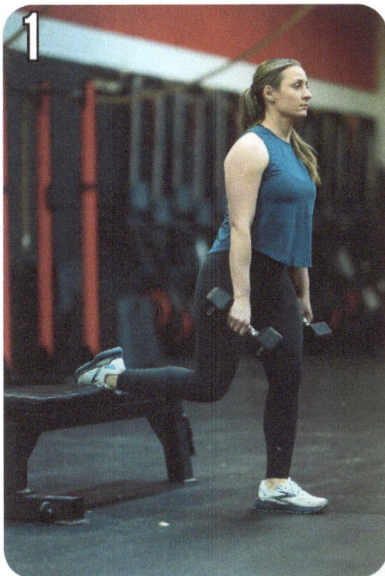

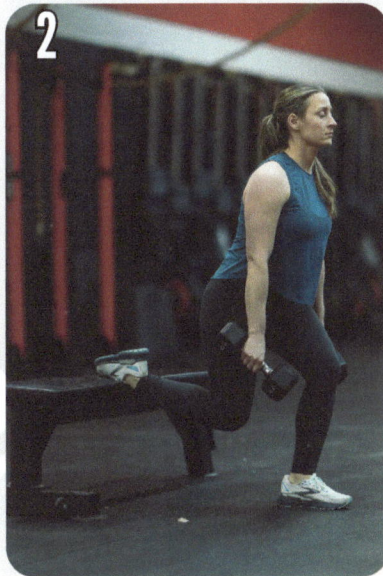

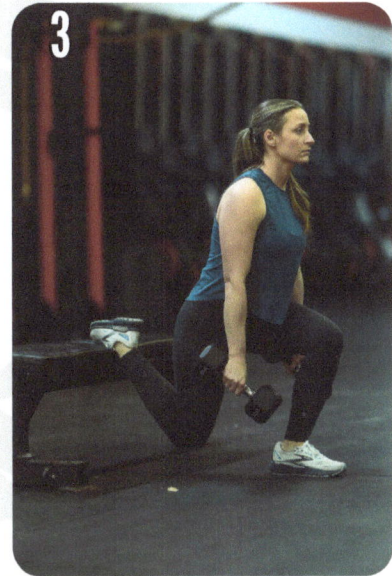

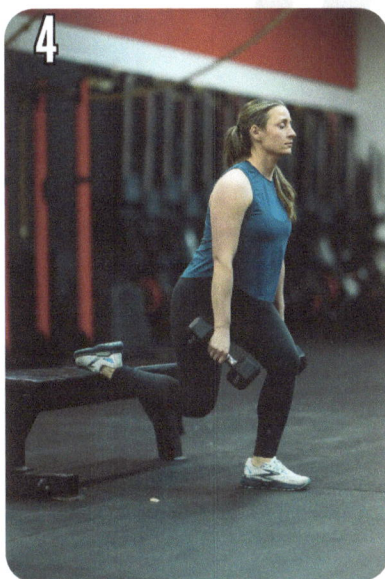

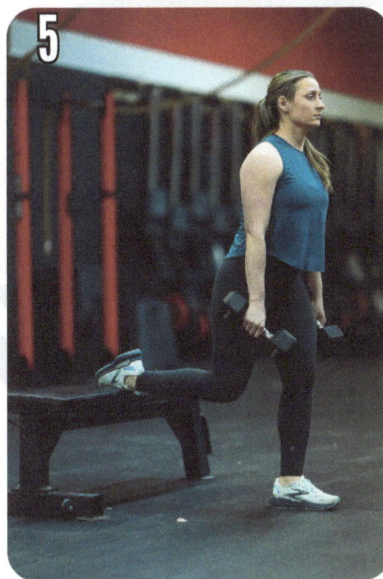

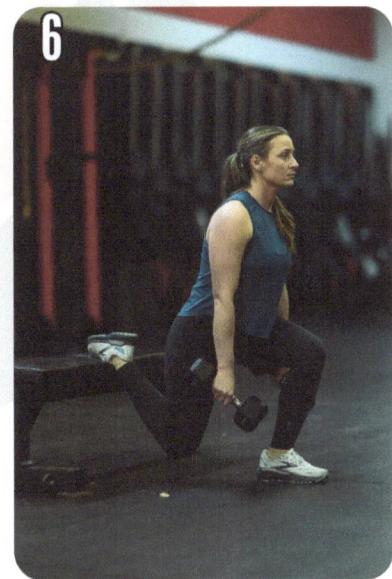

Movement Appendix
Bodyweight Variations

Hanging Knee Raises

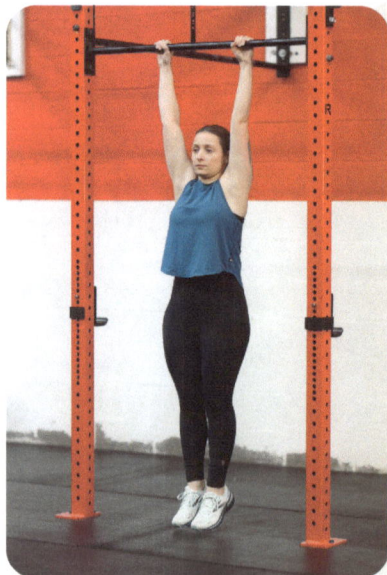 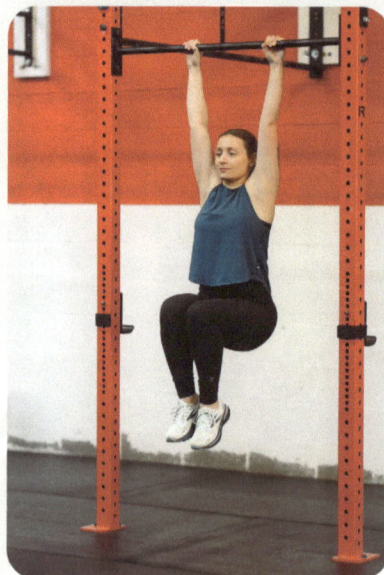 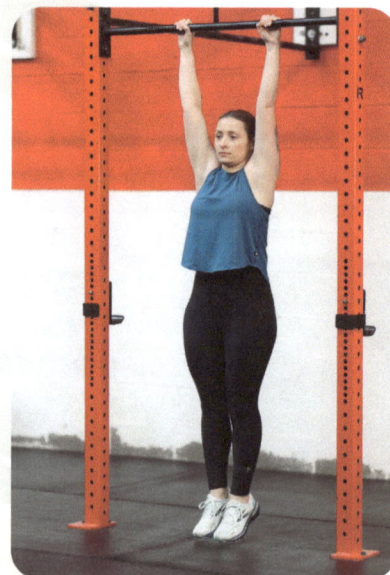

Pull ups   **Chin Ups**   **L-Sits**

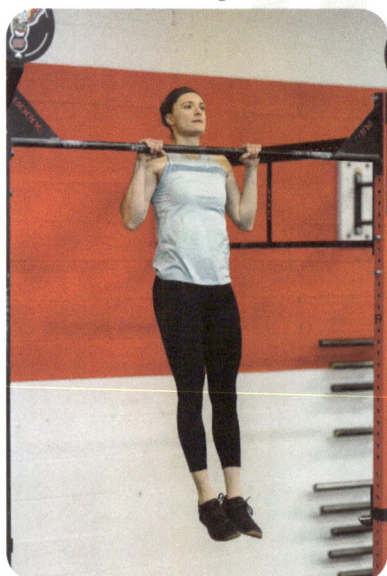 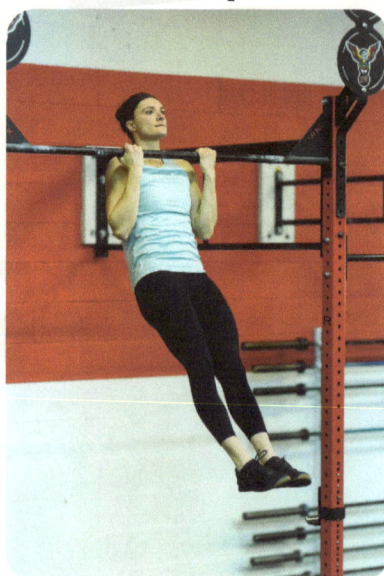 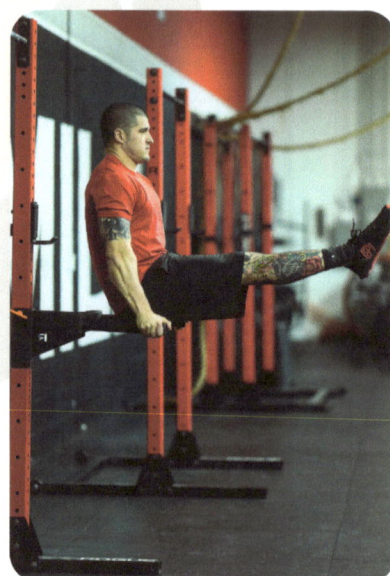

Stronger On Scene

Movement Appendix
Bodyweight Variations

V-Ups

1-Leg V-Ups

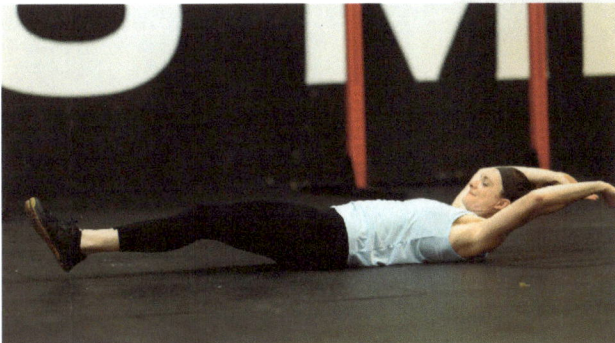
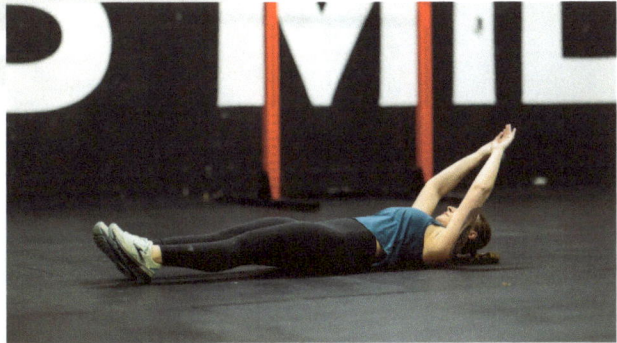
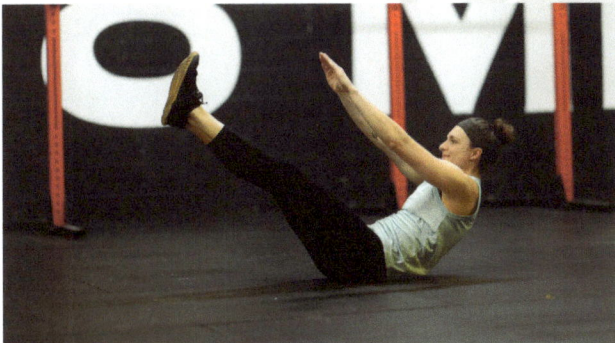
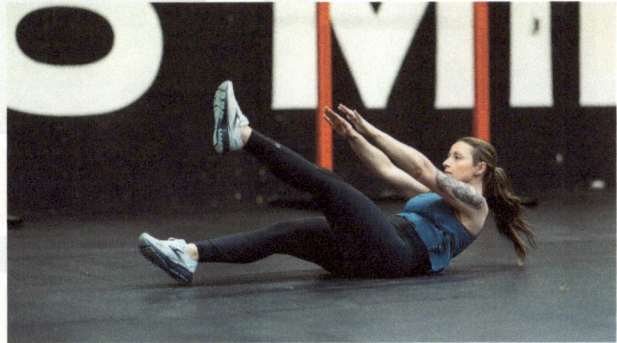
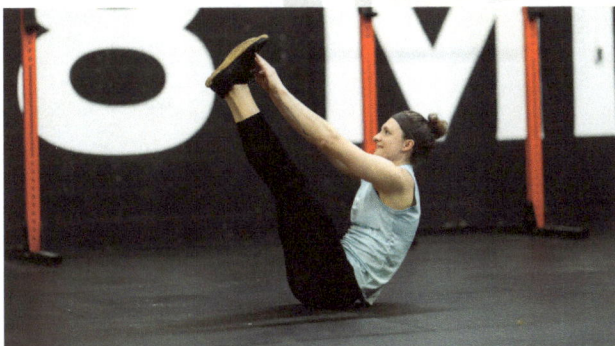
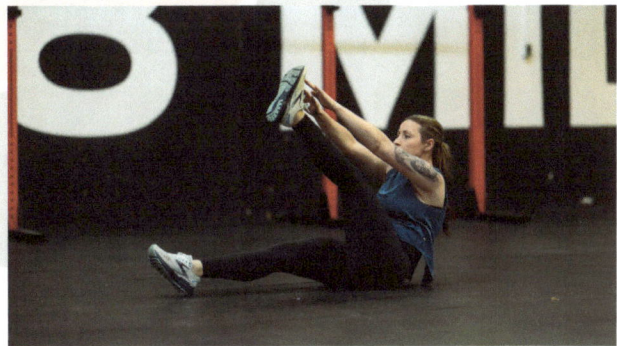

Movement Appendix
Bodyweight Variations

Deficit Push Ups

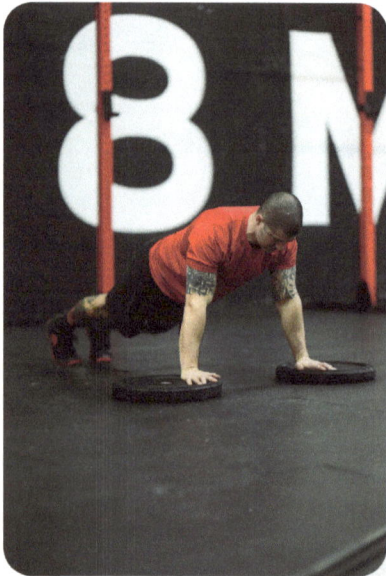

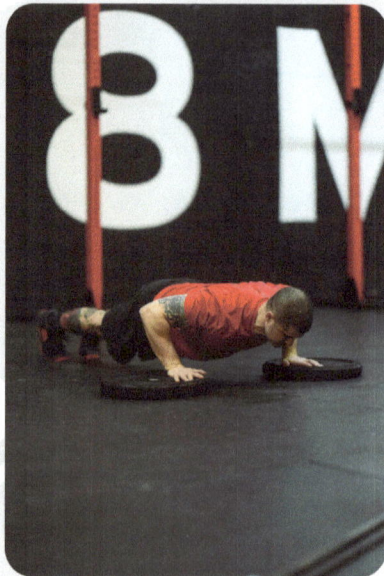

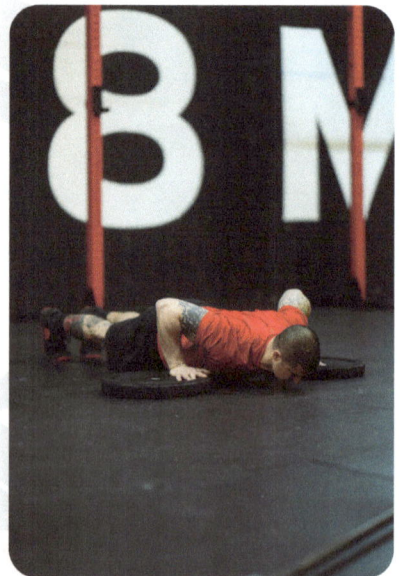

Burpees Over Barrier

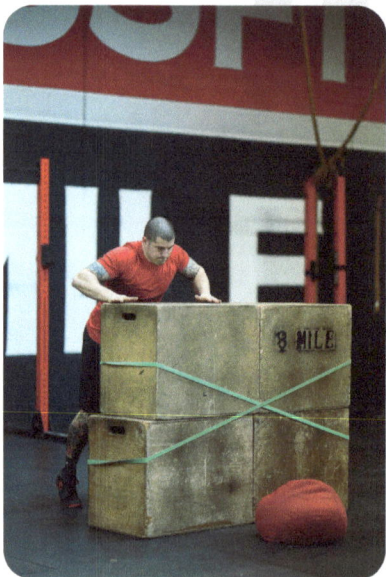

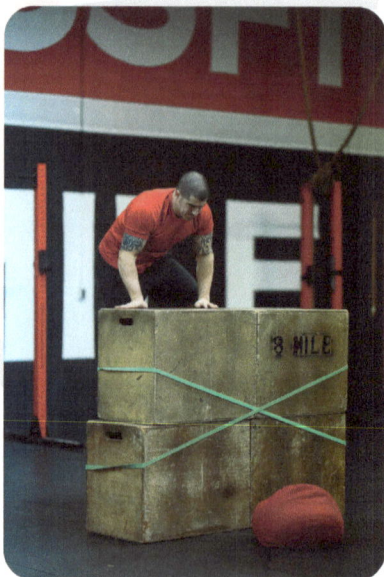

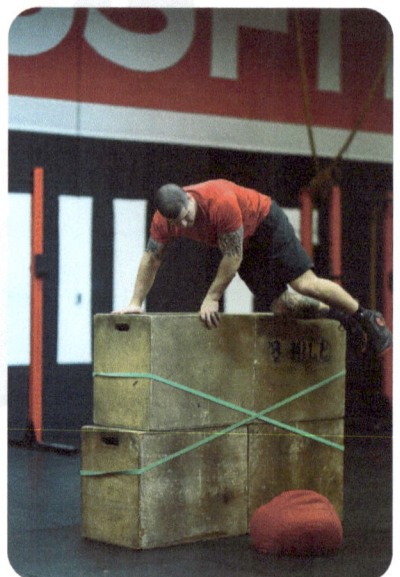

Movement Appendix
Hinge Variations

Russian Kettlebell Swings

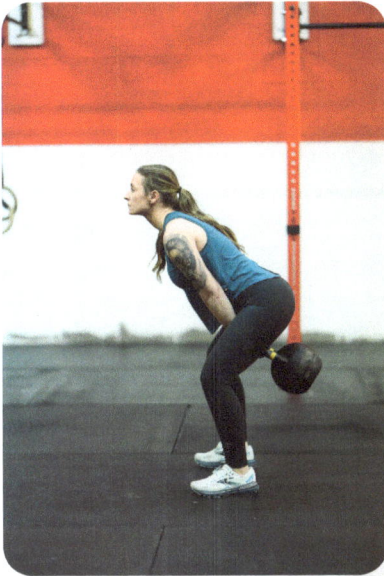 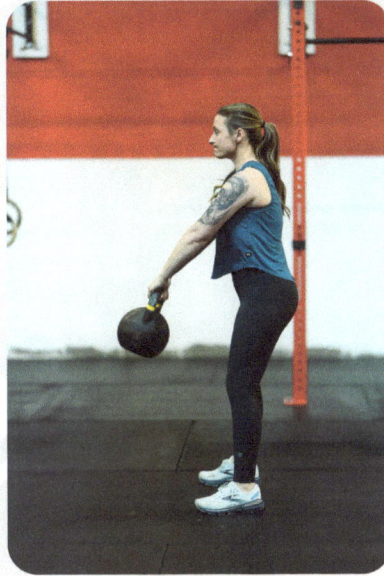 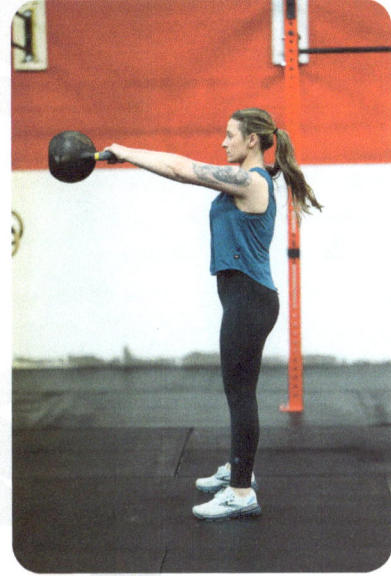

Deadlifts

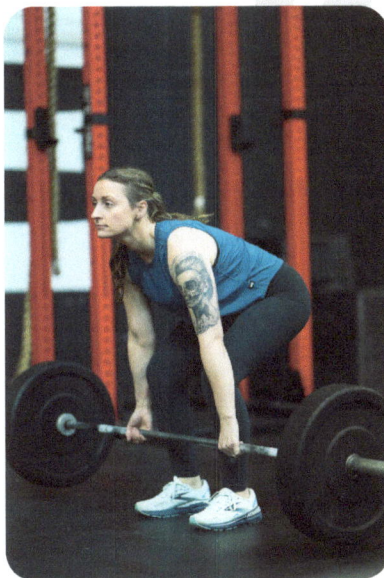 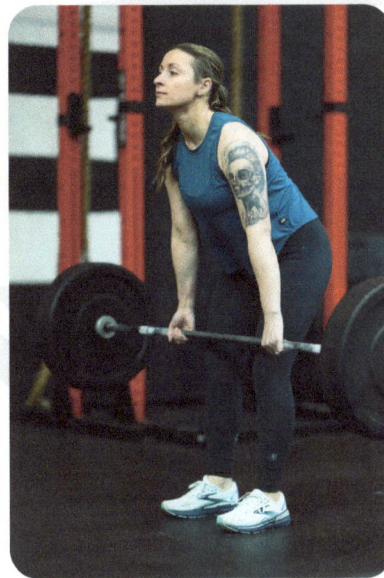 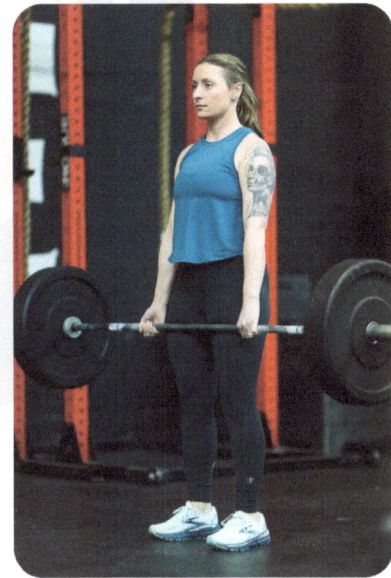

Movement Appendix
Hinge Variations

Front Rack Kettlebell Lunges

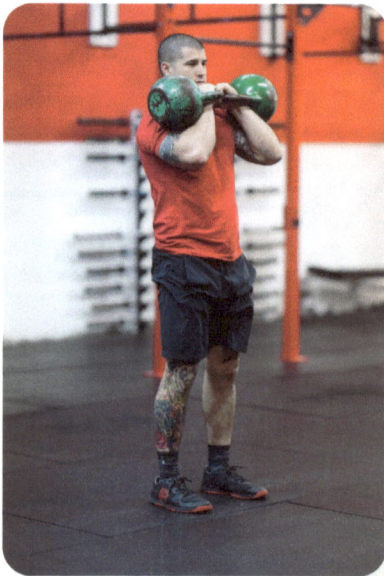

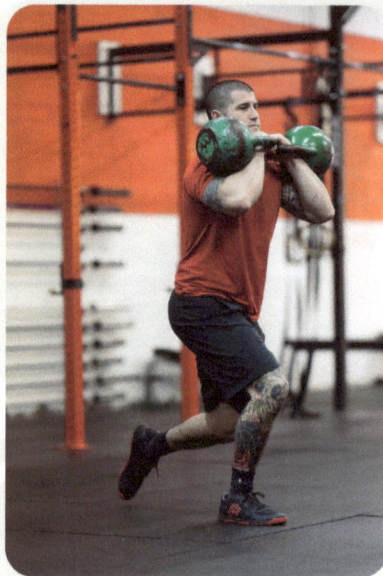

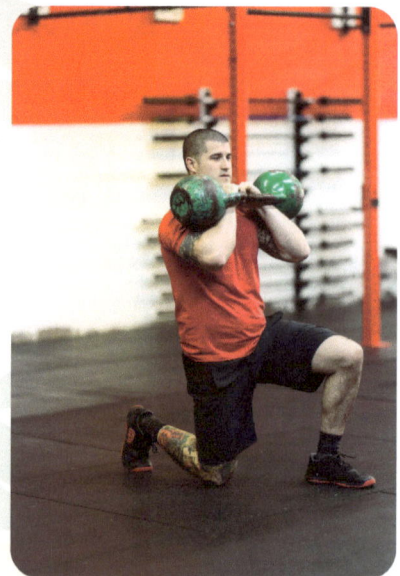

Back Rack Lunges

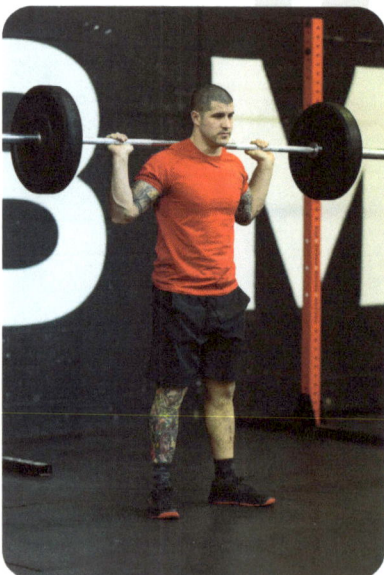

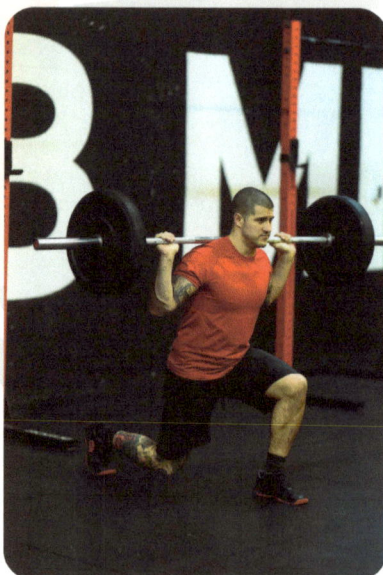

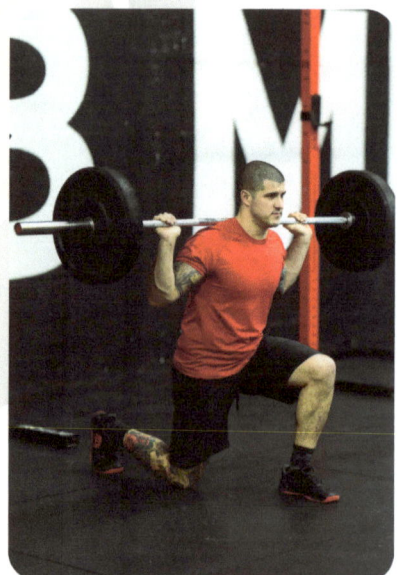

Movement Appendix
Hinge Variations

Dumbbell Dimmel Deadlift

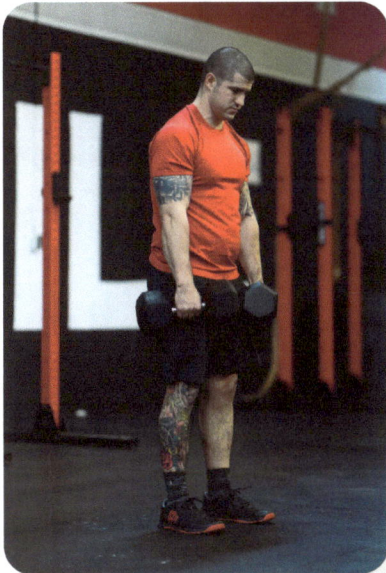

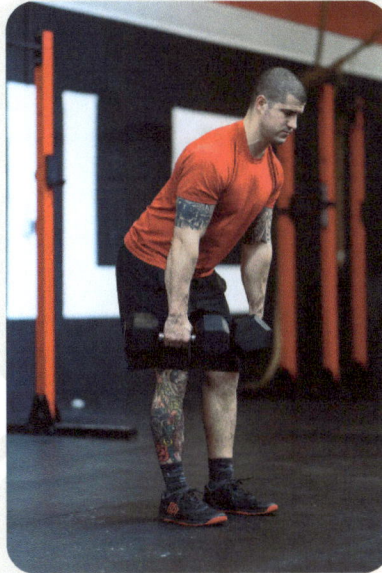

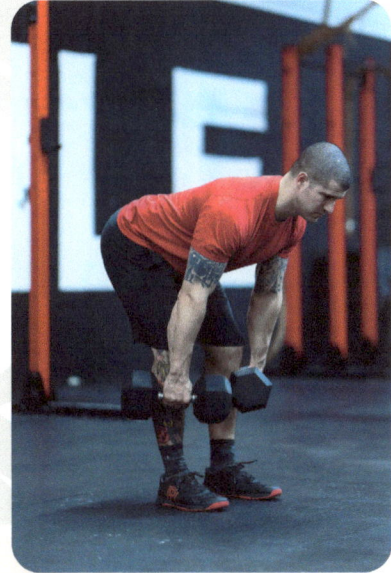

Explosive Kettlebell Deadlifts

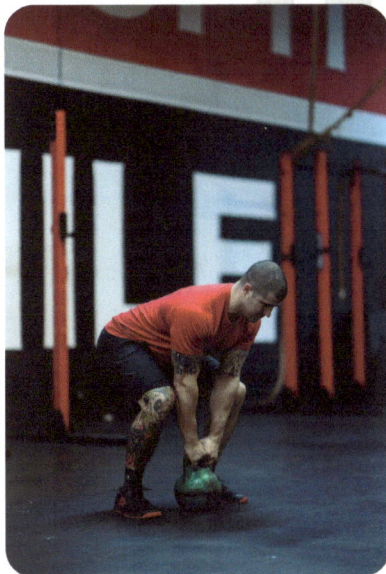

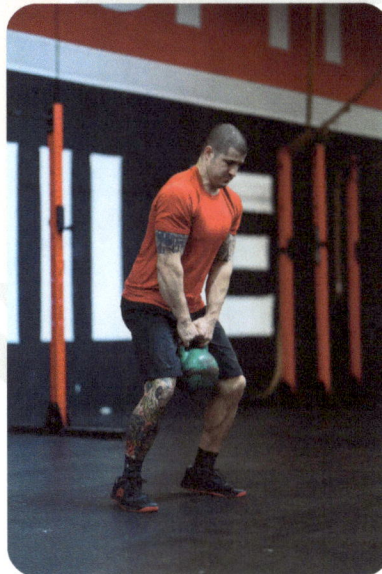

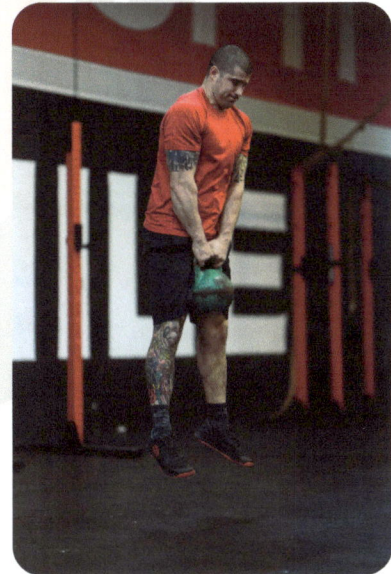

Stronger On Scene

Movement Appendix
Clean Variations

Barbell Power Clean

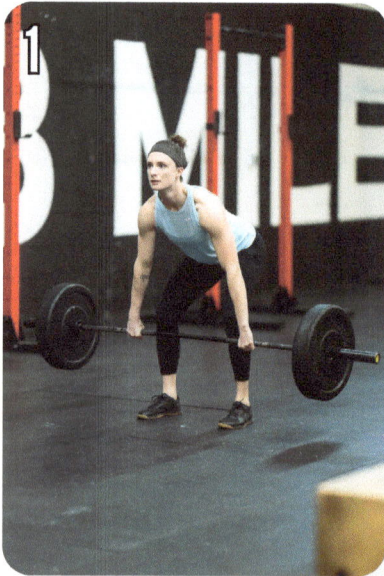

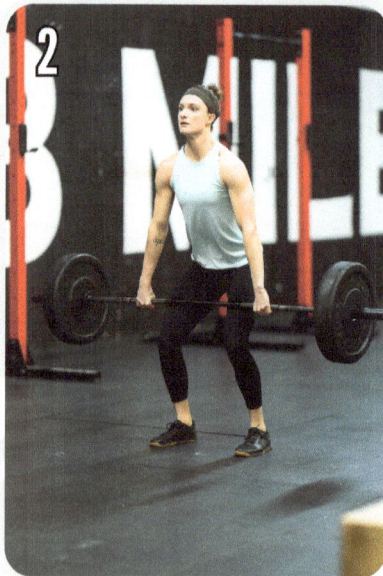

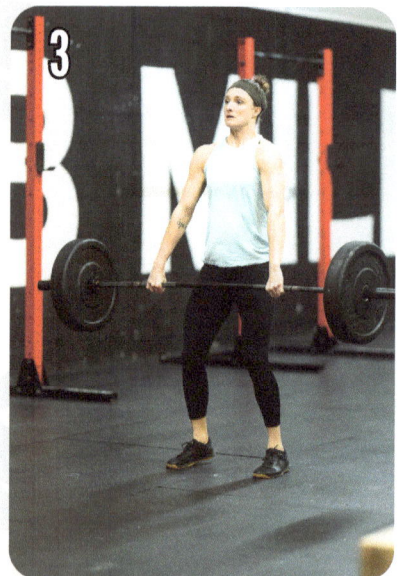

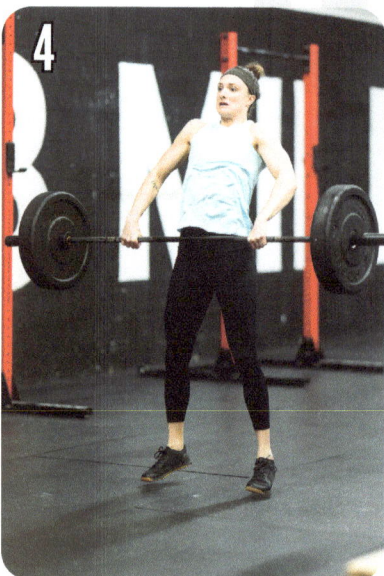

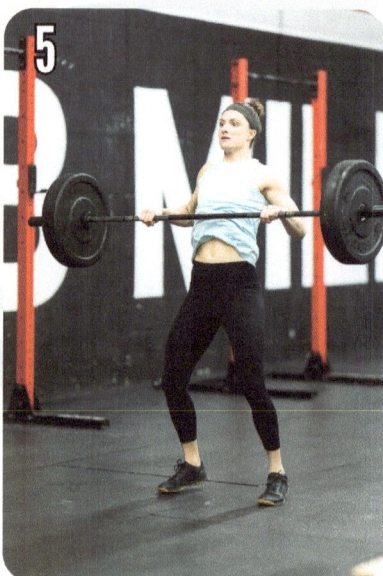

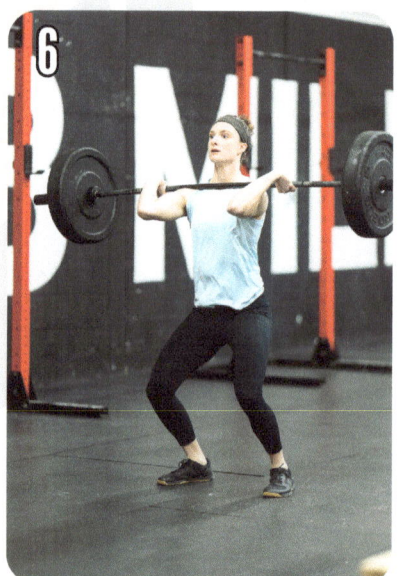

Movement Appendix
Clean Variations

Double Kettlebell Clean

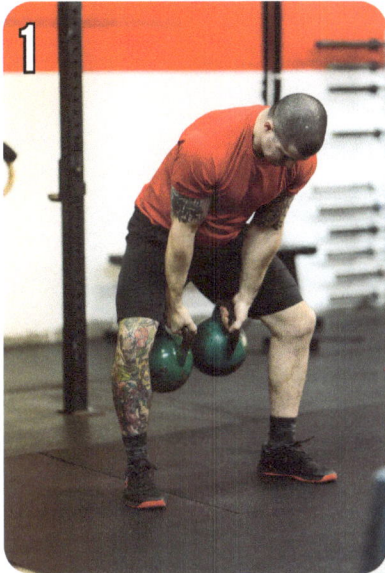

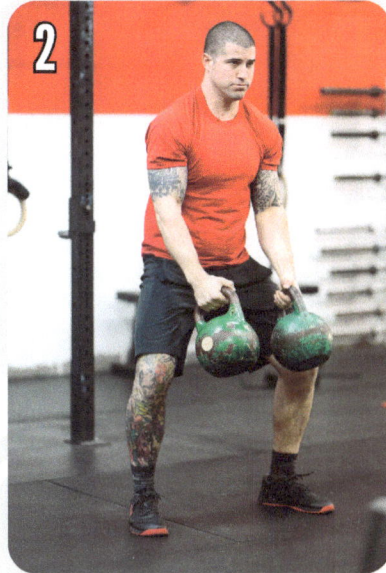

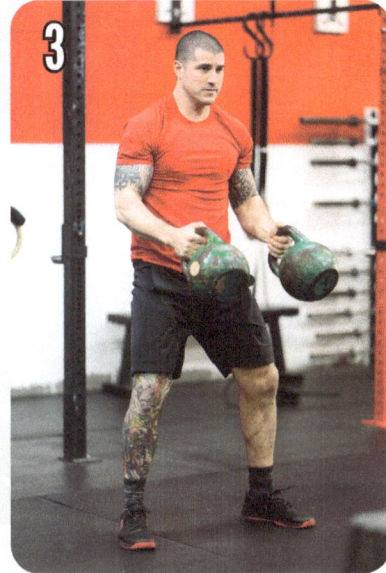

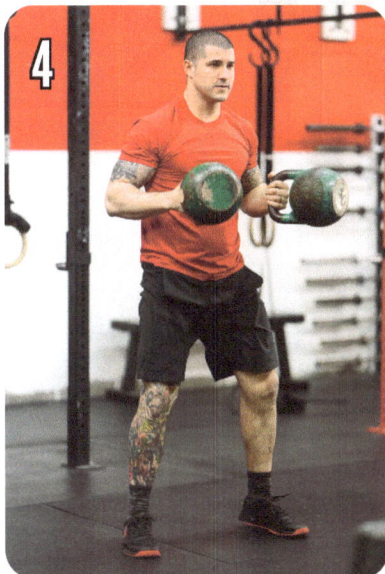

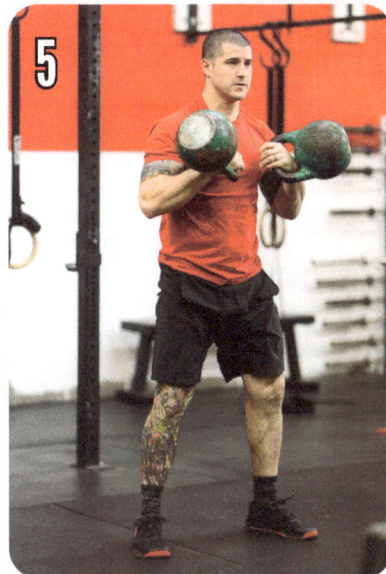

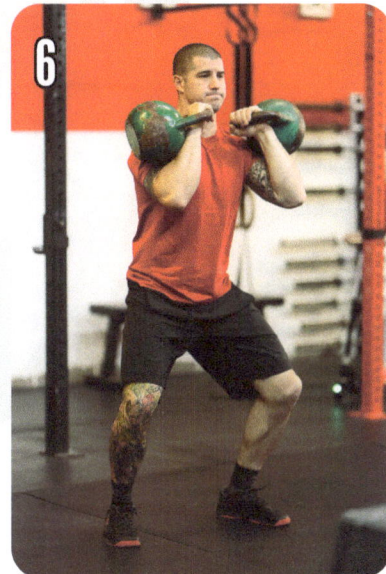

Movement Appendix
Clean Variations

Double Dumbbell Clean

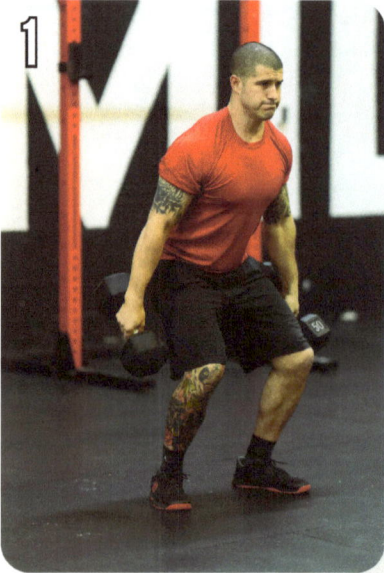

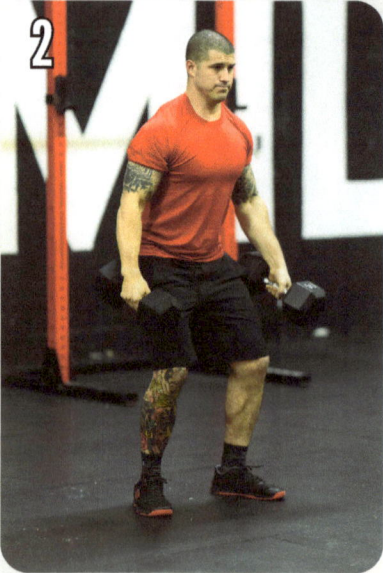

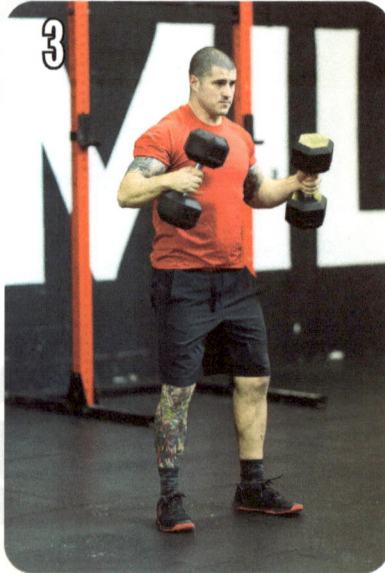

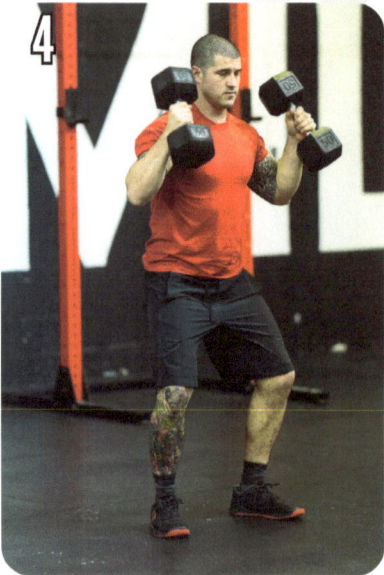

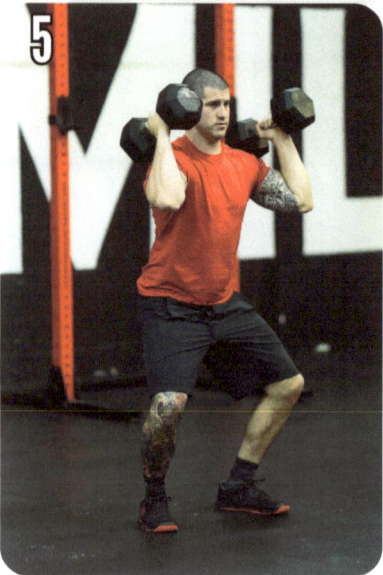

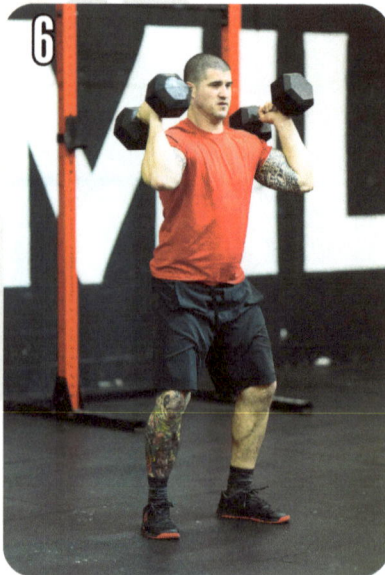

Movement Appendix
Clean Variations

Sandbag Clean

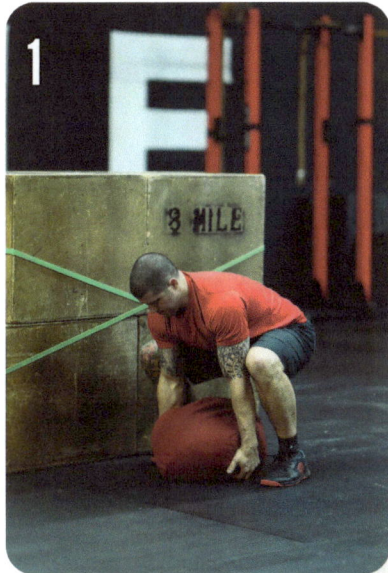

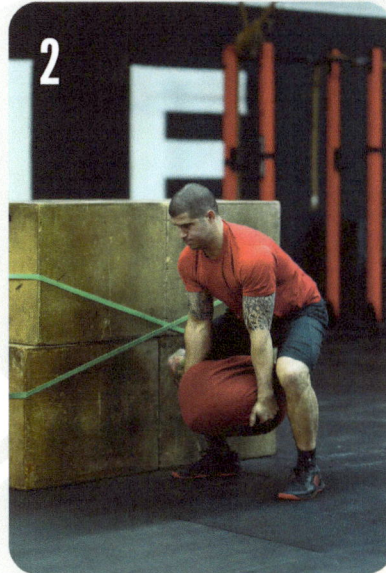

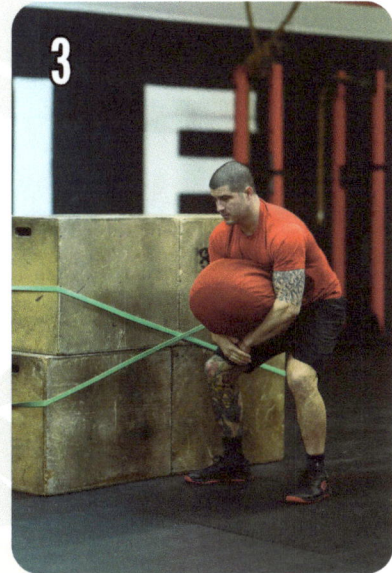

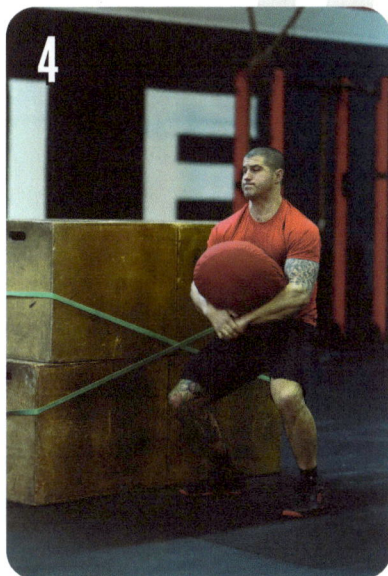

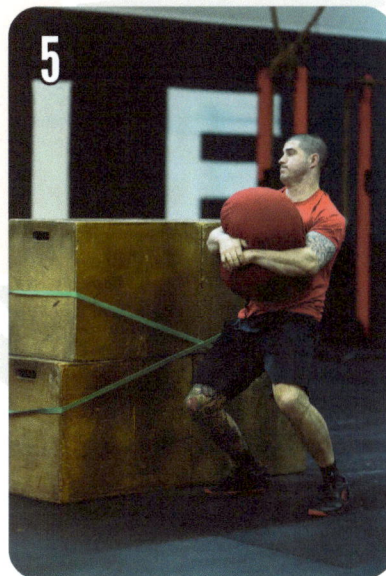

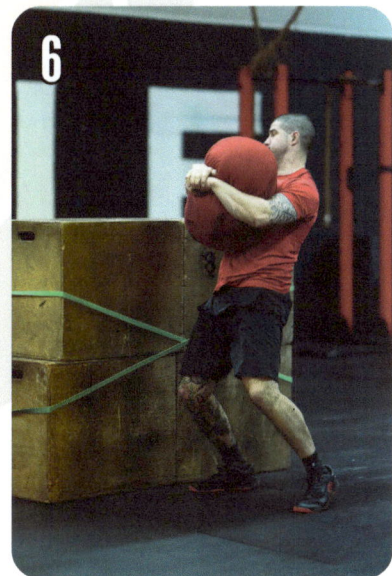

Movement Appendix
Push/Pull Variations

Strict Press

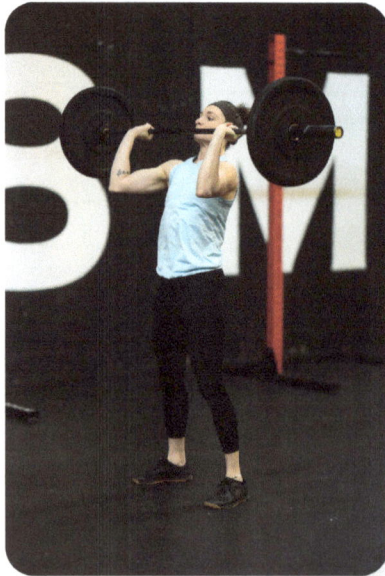

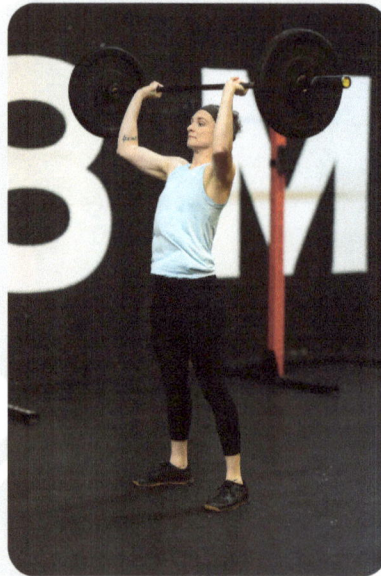

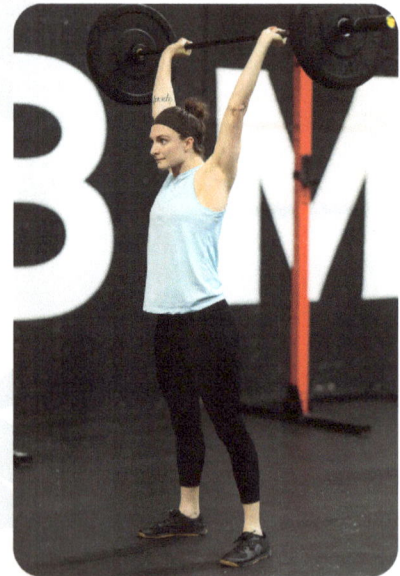

Single Arm Kettlebell Press

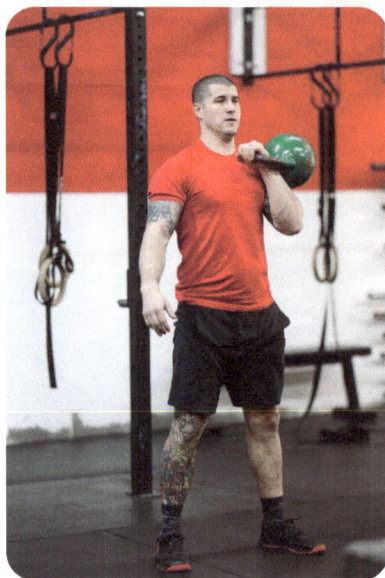

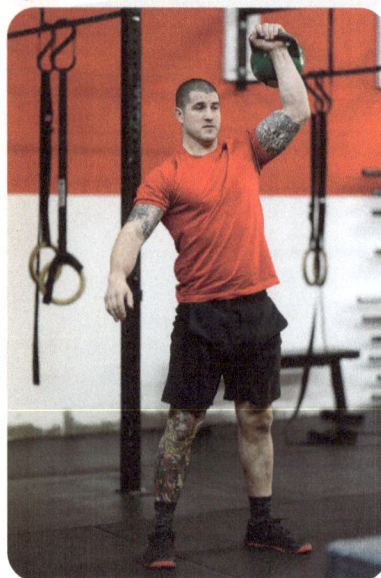

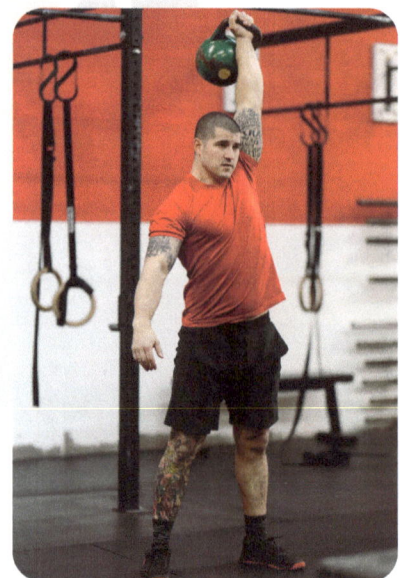

Stronger On Scene

Movement Appendix
Push/Pull Variations

Alternating Kettlebell Press

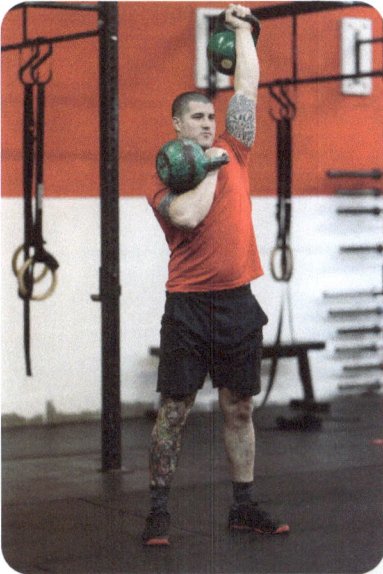

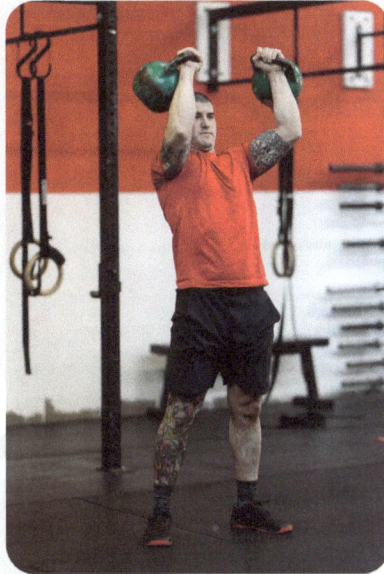

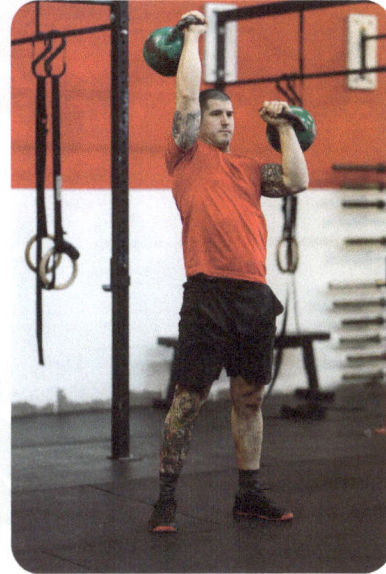

Dumbbell Push Press

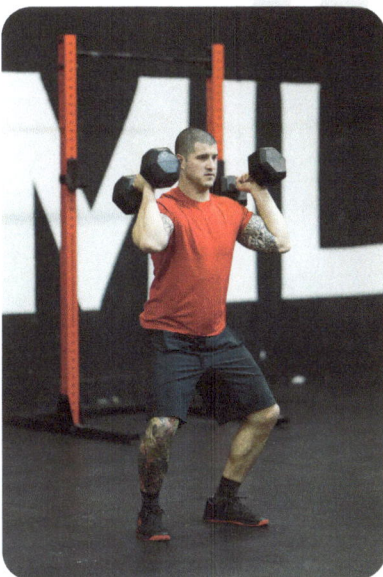

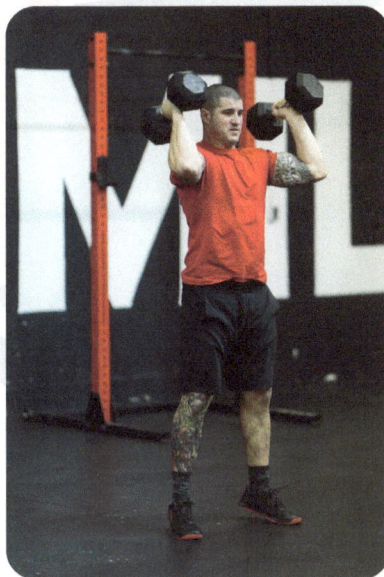

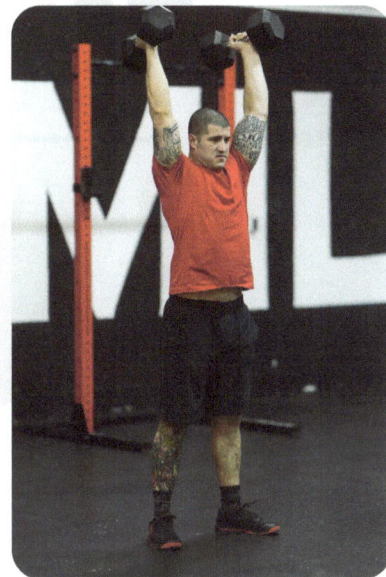

Stronger On Scene

Movement Appendix
Push/Pull Variations

Dumbbell Snatch

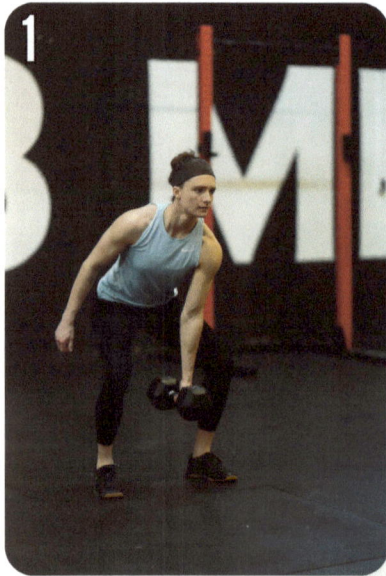

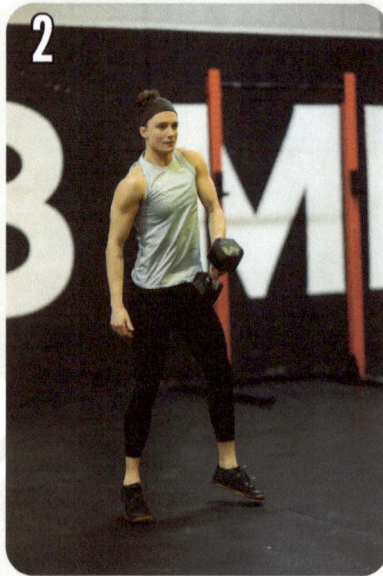

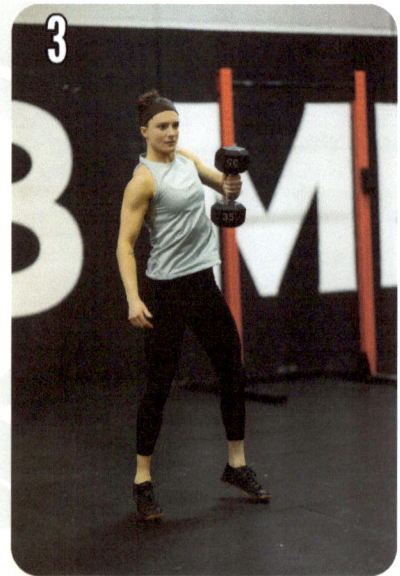

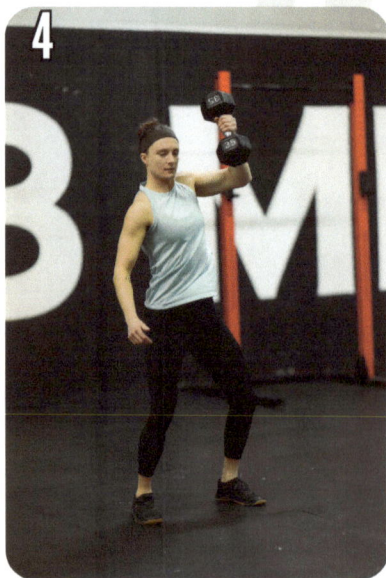

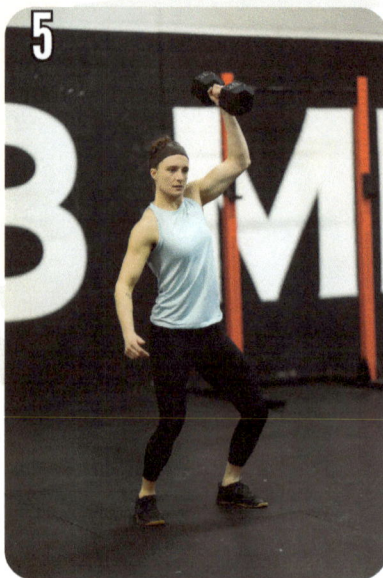

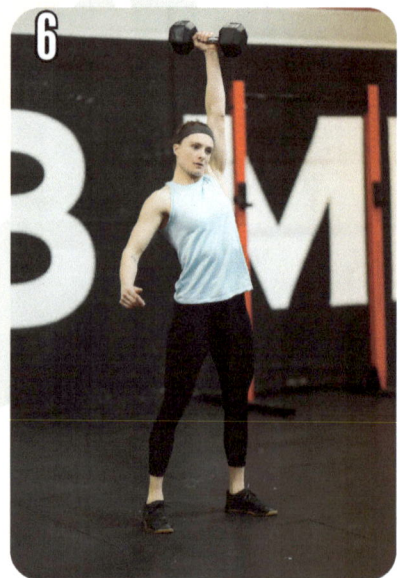

Movement Appendix
Push/Pull Variations

Kettlebell Snatch

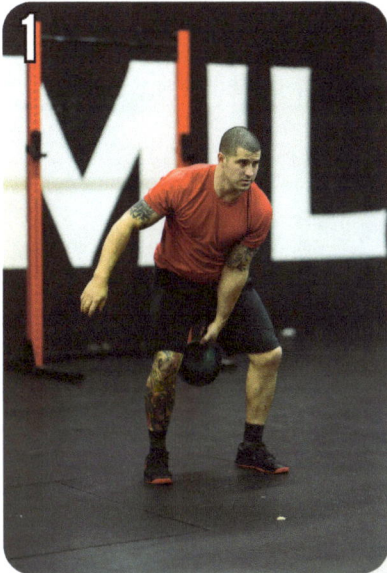

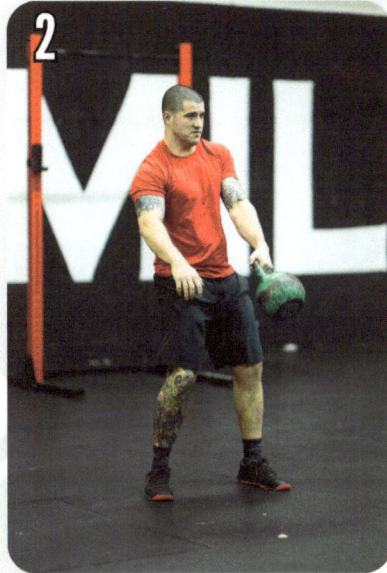

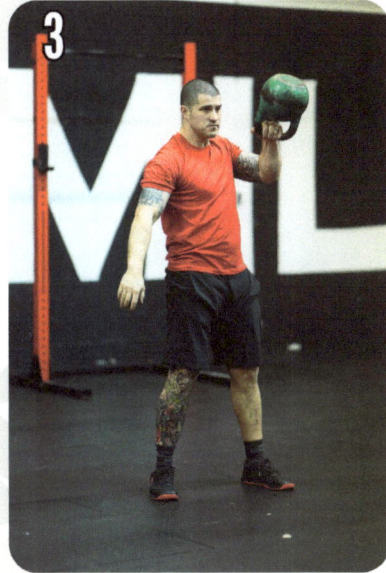

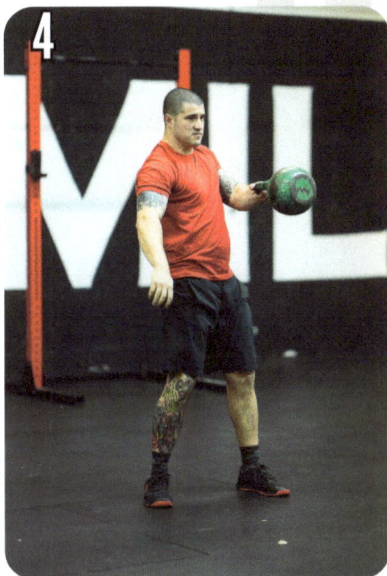

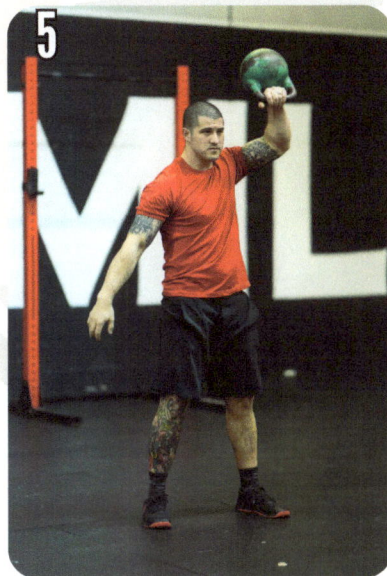

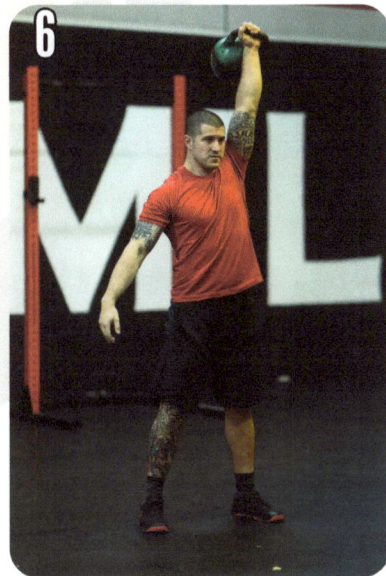

Movement Appendix
Push/Pull Variations

Kettlebell Push Jerk

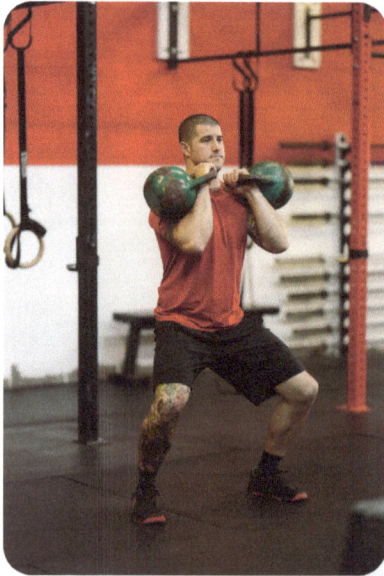

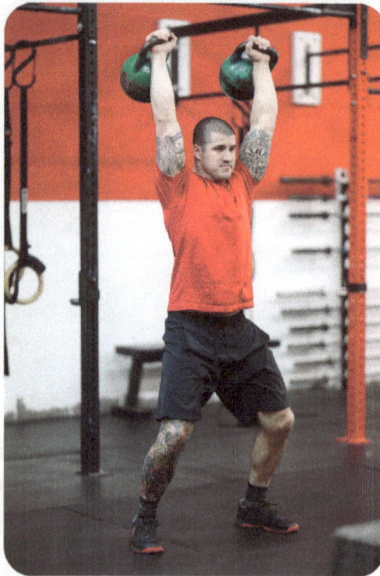

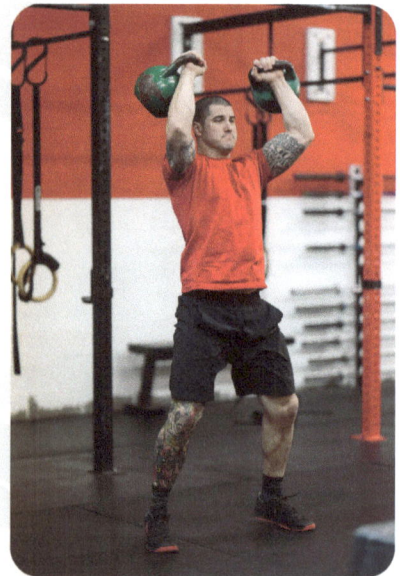

Dumbbell Upright Row

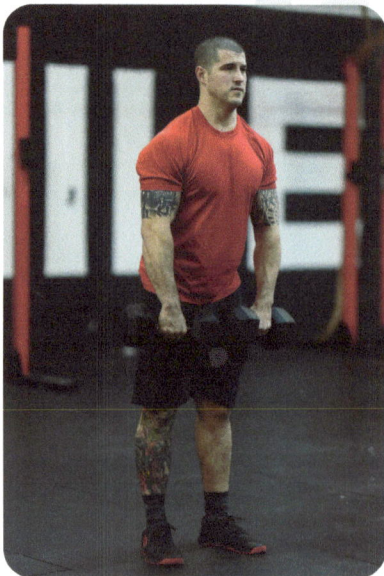

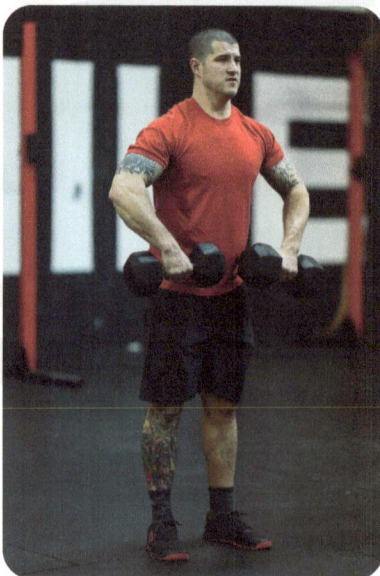

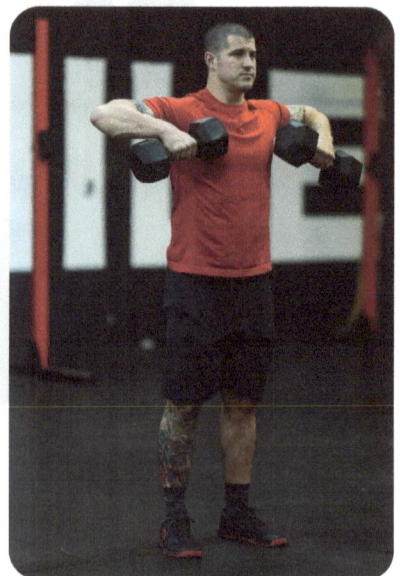

Stronger On Scene

Movement Appendix
Push/Pull Variations

Double Dumbbell Bent Over Row

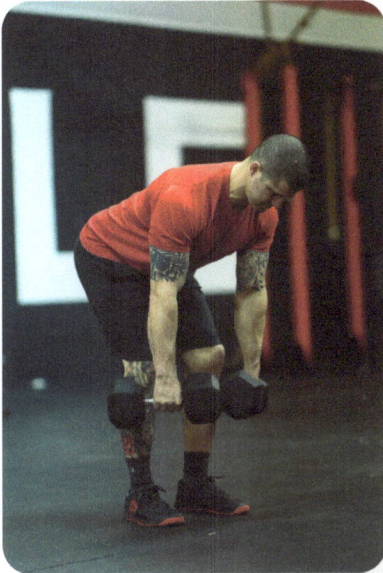

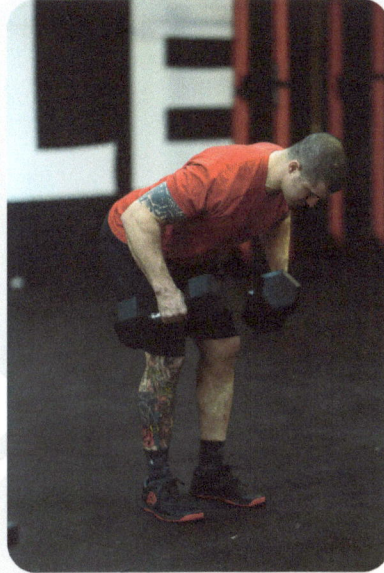

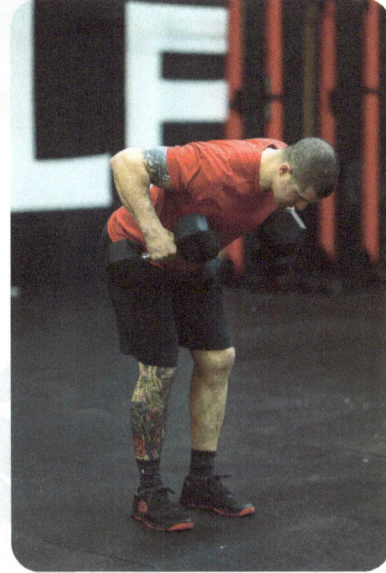

1-Arm Dumbbell Row

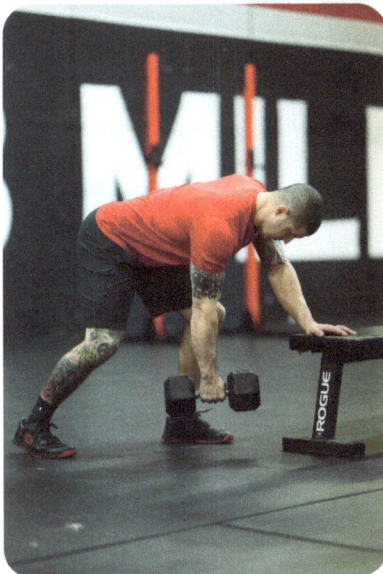

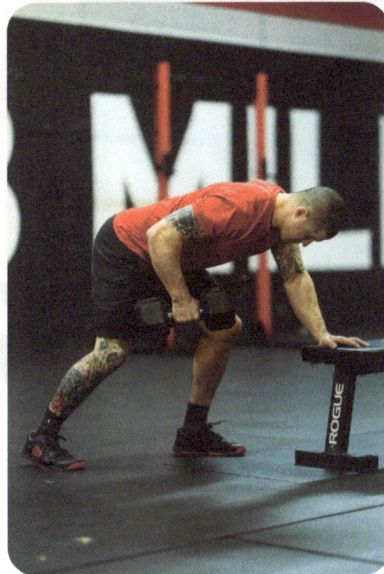

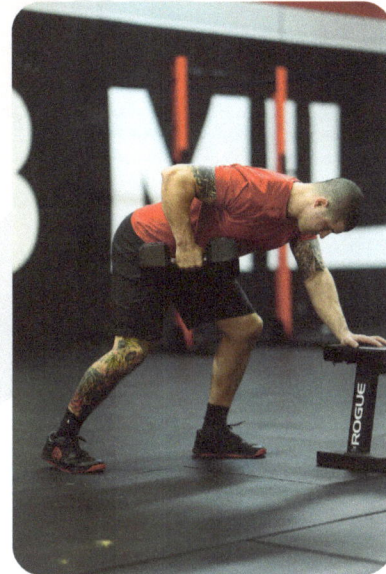

Stronger On Scene

Movement Appendix
Push/Pull Variations

Renegade Rows

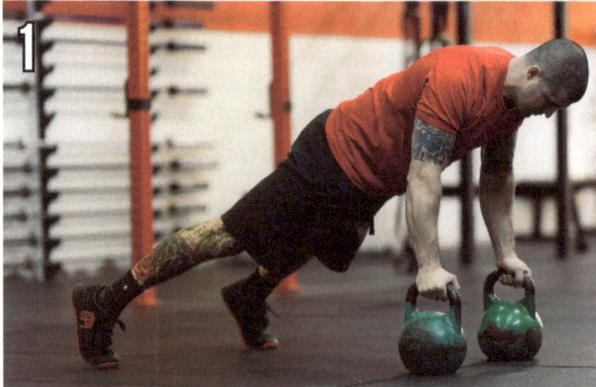

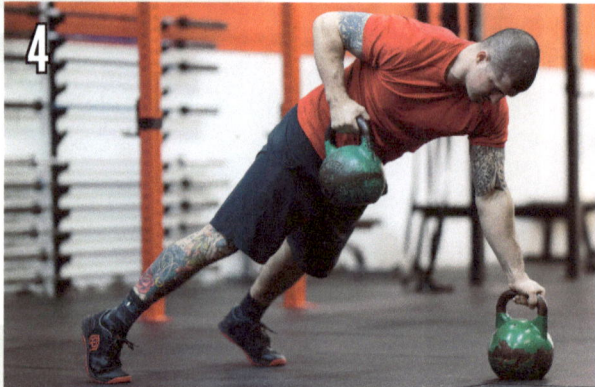

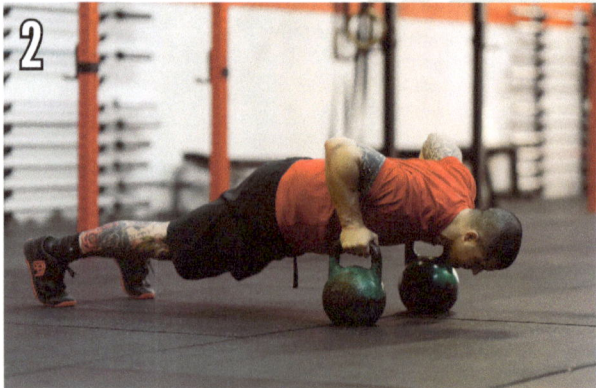

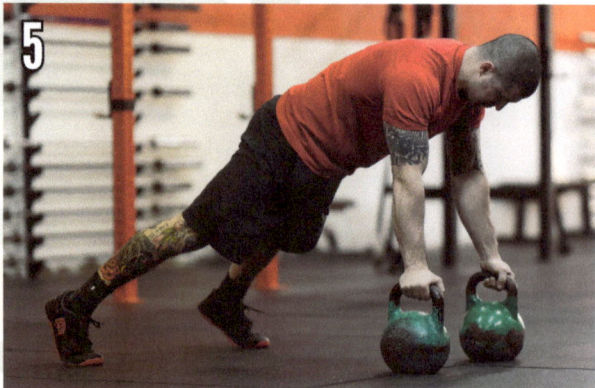

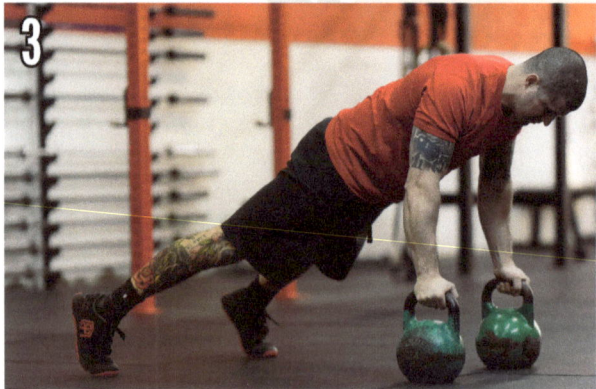

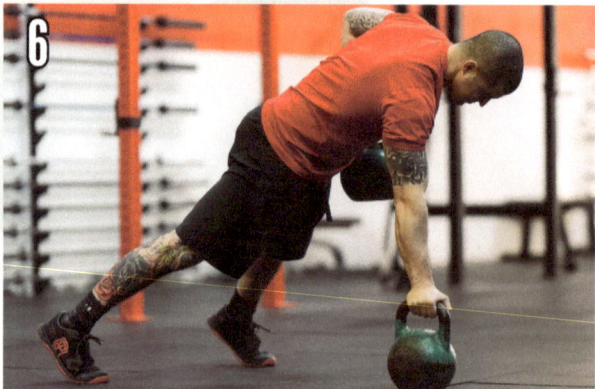

Movement Appendix
Miscellaneous

Sled Push

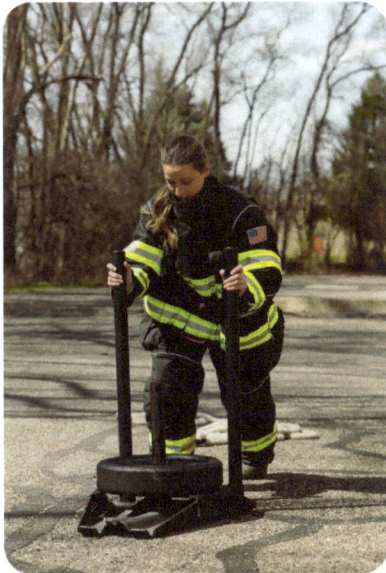

Sled Drag Forward

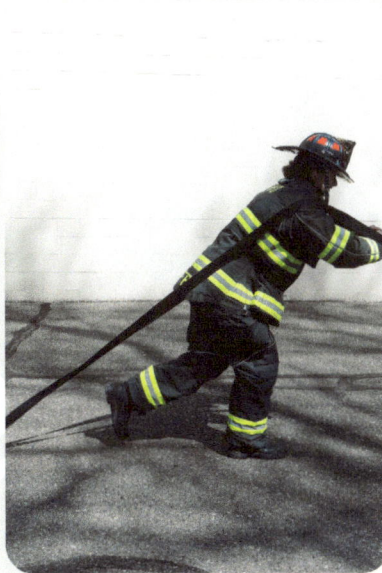

Sled Drag Backward

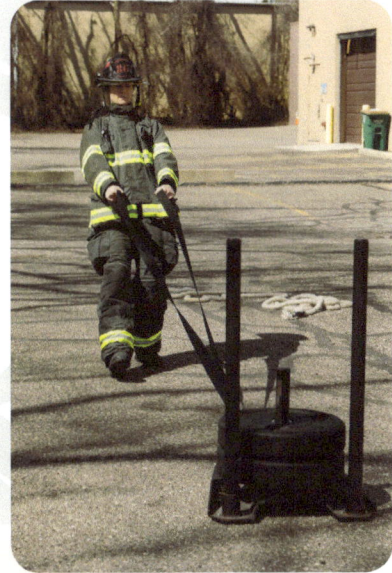

HOH Sled Pull

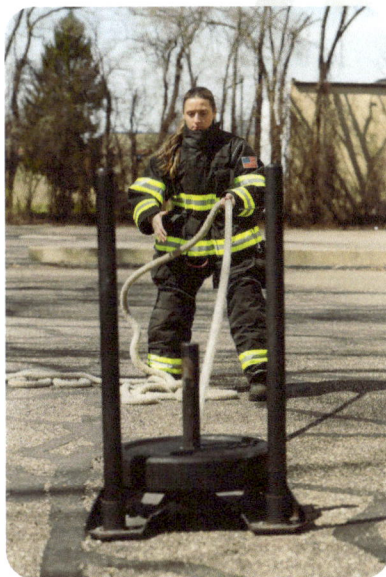

Sledge Strikes

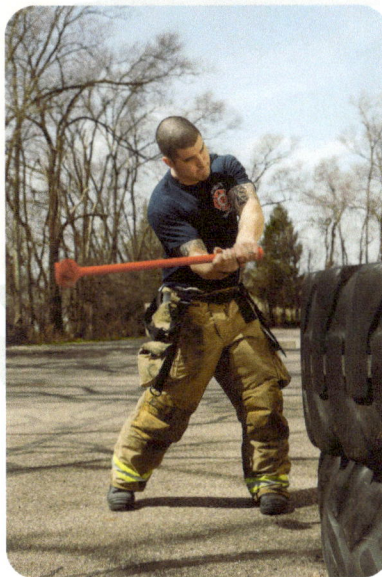

Stair Stepper

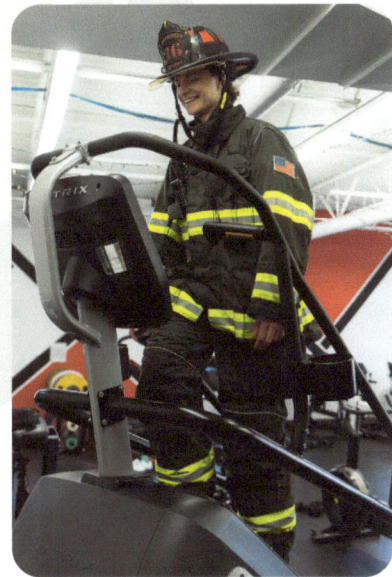

Stronger On Scene

Movement Appendix
Miscellaneous

Dumbbell Pull Throughs

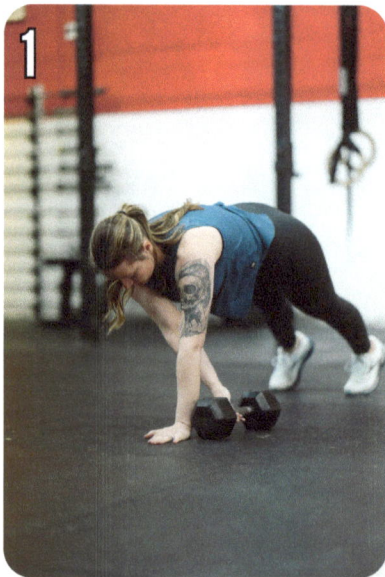

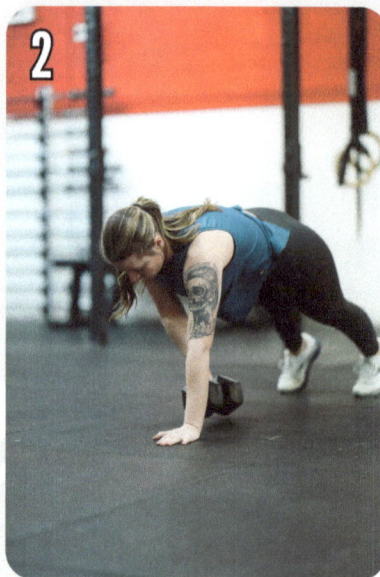

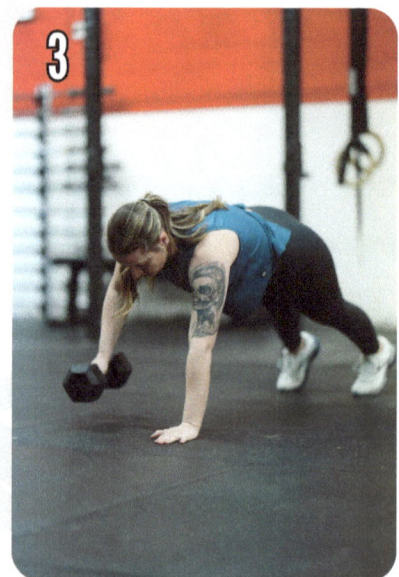

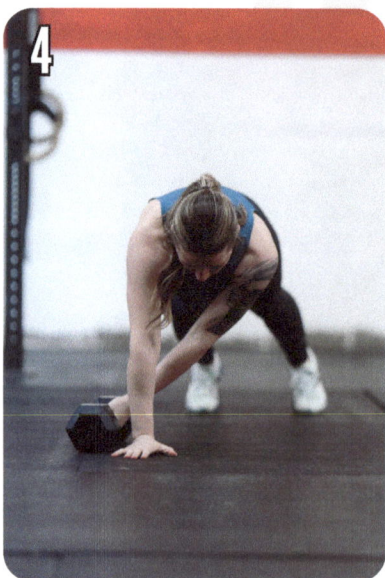

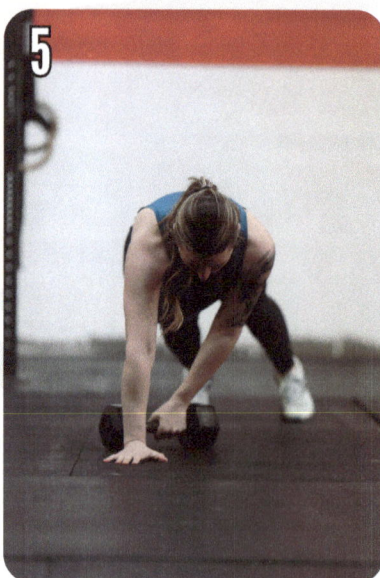

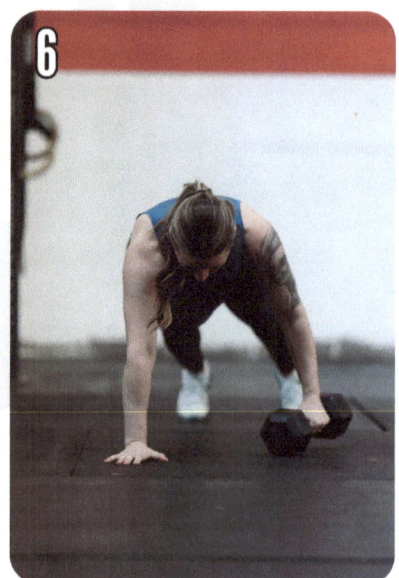

Stronger On Scene

Movement Appendix
Miscellaneous

Sandbag Over Barrier

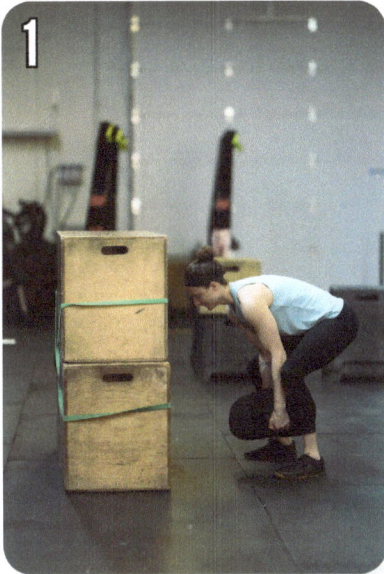

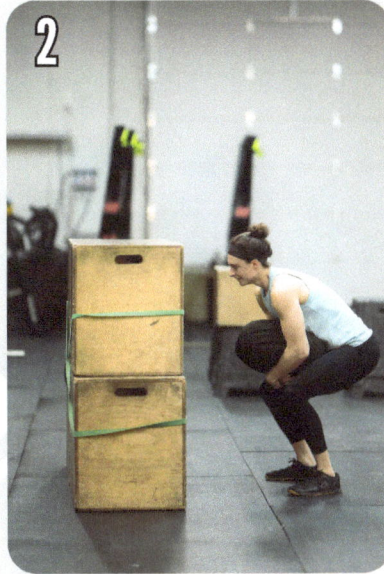

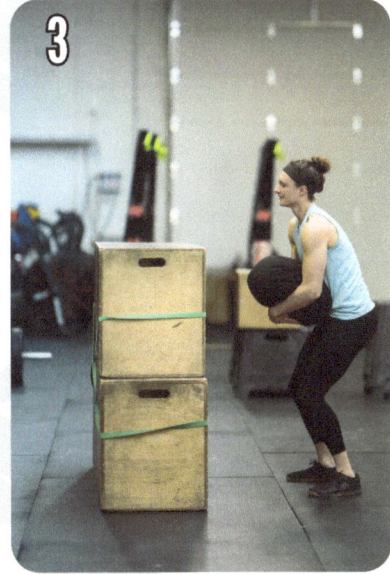

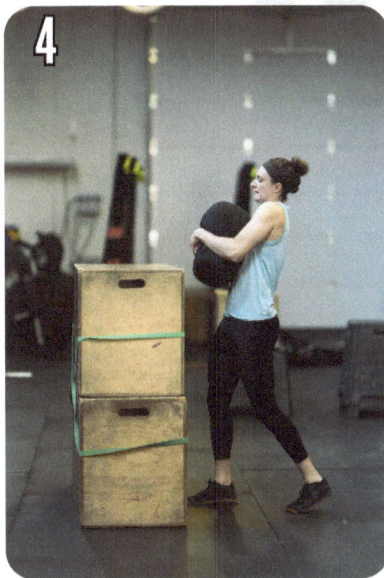

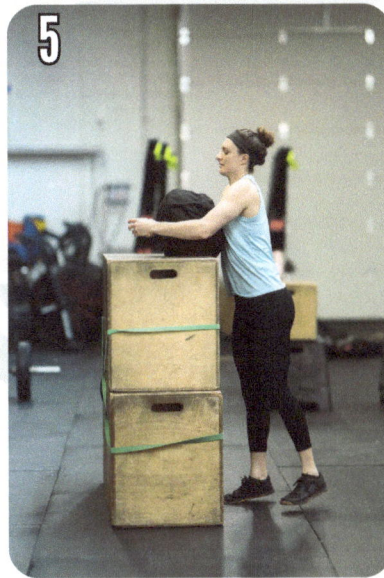

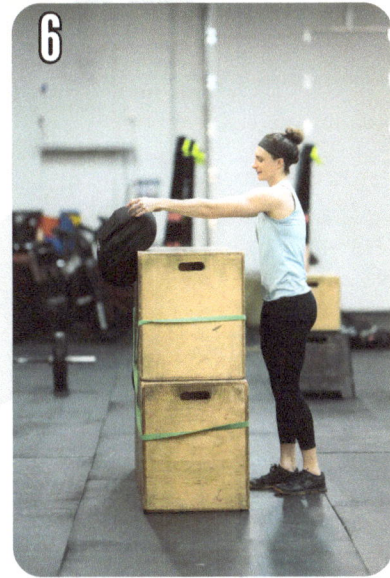

Movement Appendix
Miscellaneous
Dumbbell Bear Crawl

Single Dumbbell

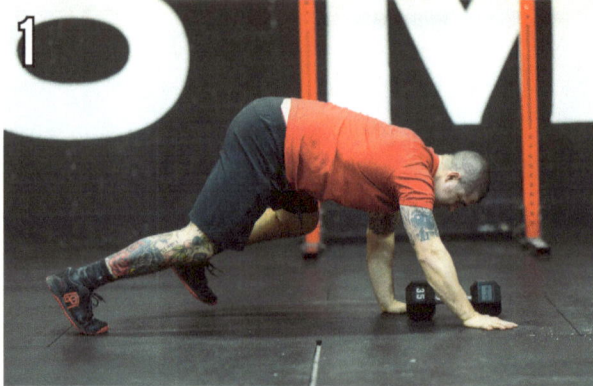

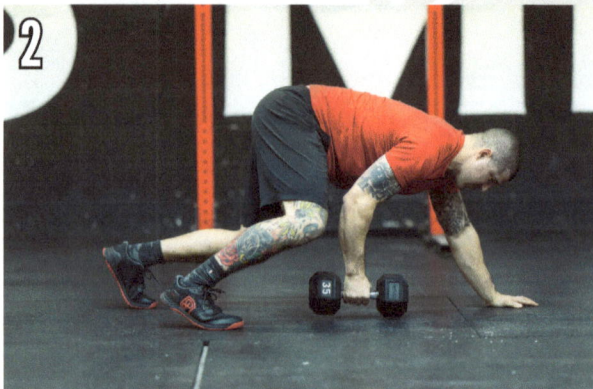

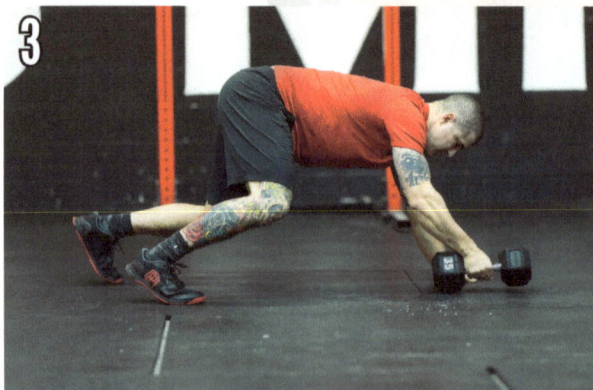

Double Dumbbell

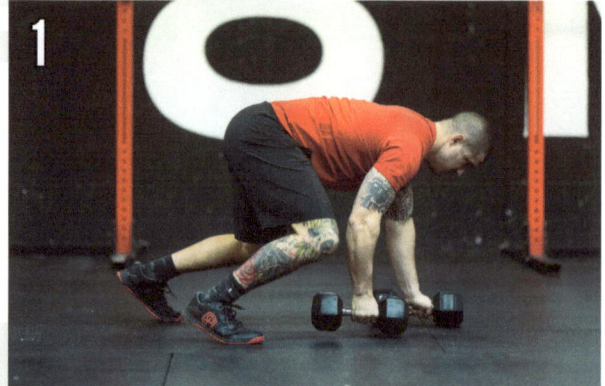

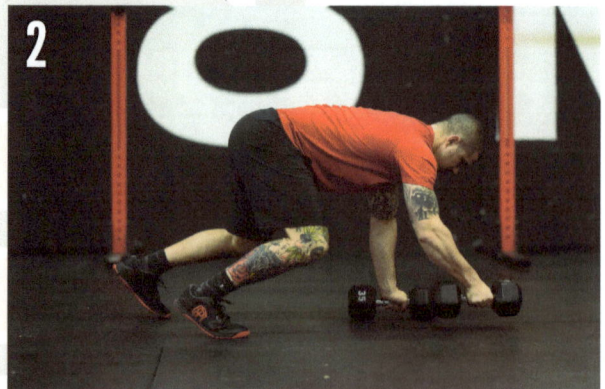

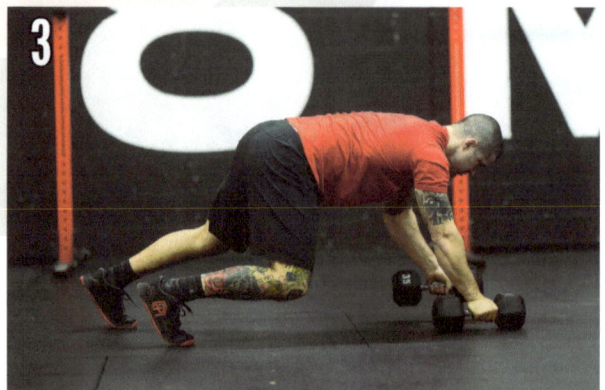

Stronger On Scene

Movement Appendix
Miscellaneous

Kneeling to Standing

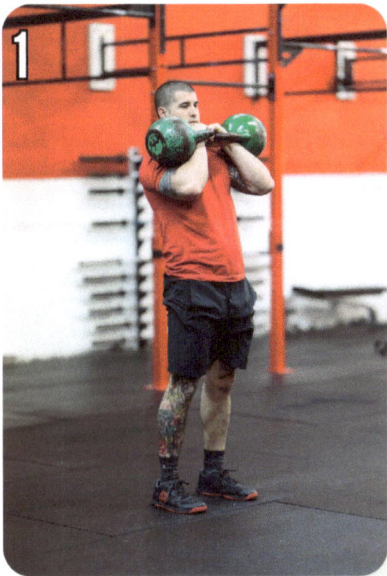

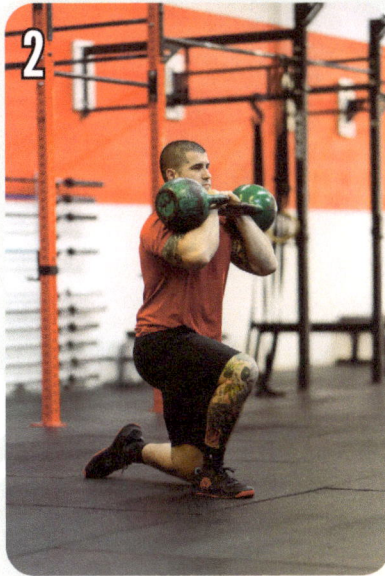

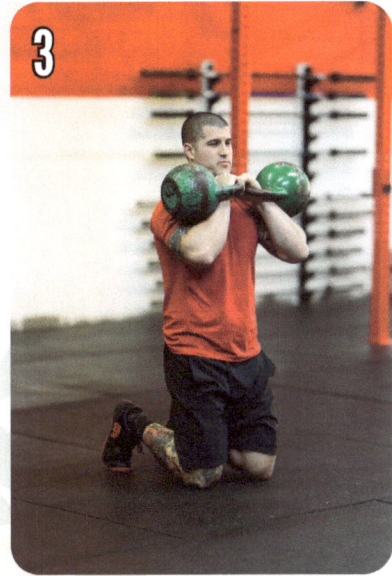

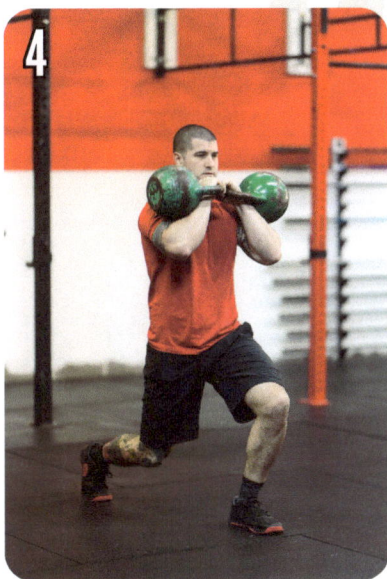

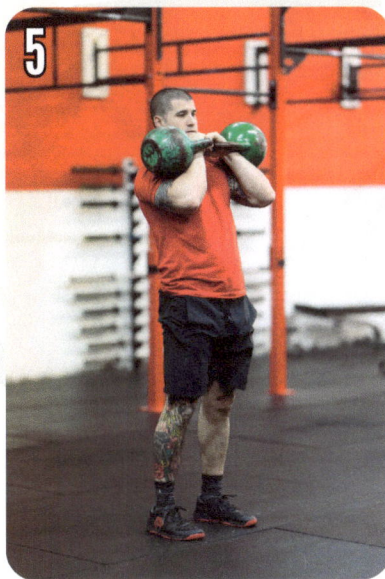

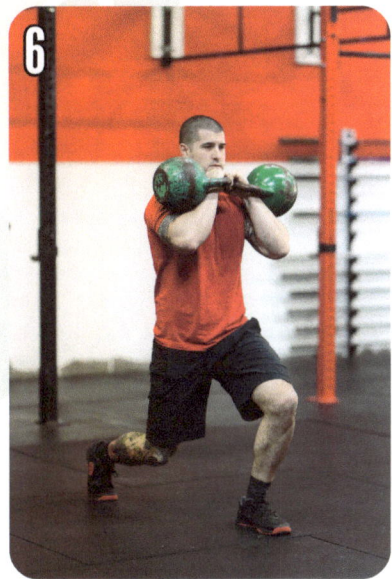

Movement Appendix
Miscellaneous

Tate Press

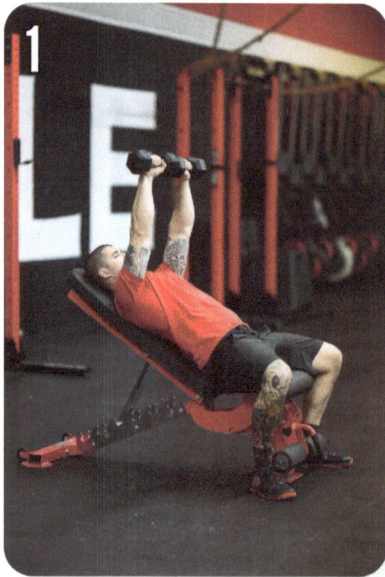 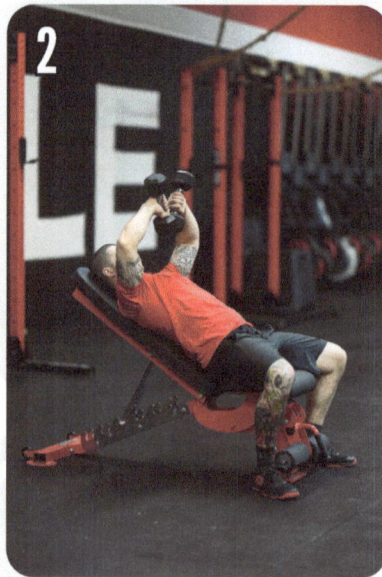 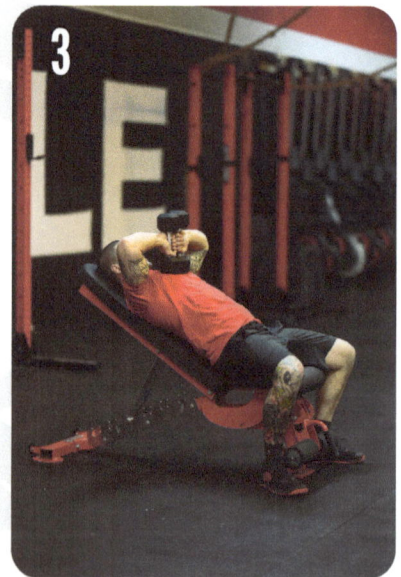

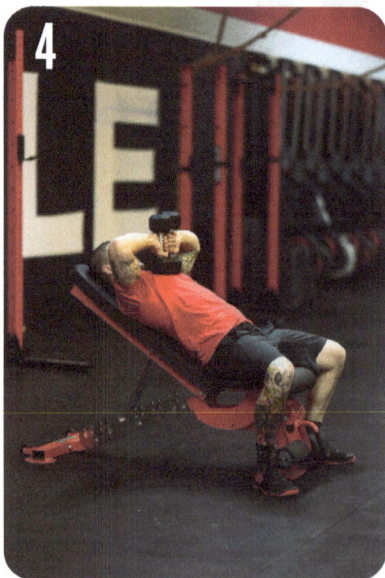 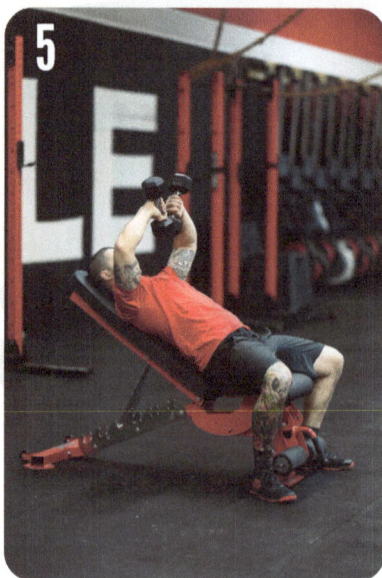 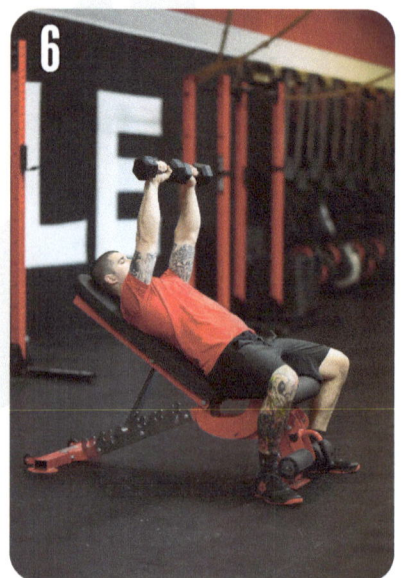

Stronger On Scene

Go to our YouTube Channel for Movement Demonstrations

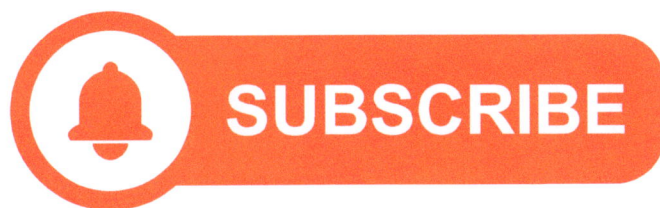

SUBSCRIBE

Stair Stepper Program

5 Levels: 24 Days of Training

CRUSH THE CPAT ONE DAY AT A TIME

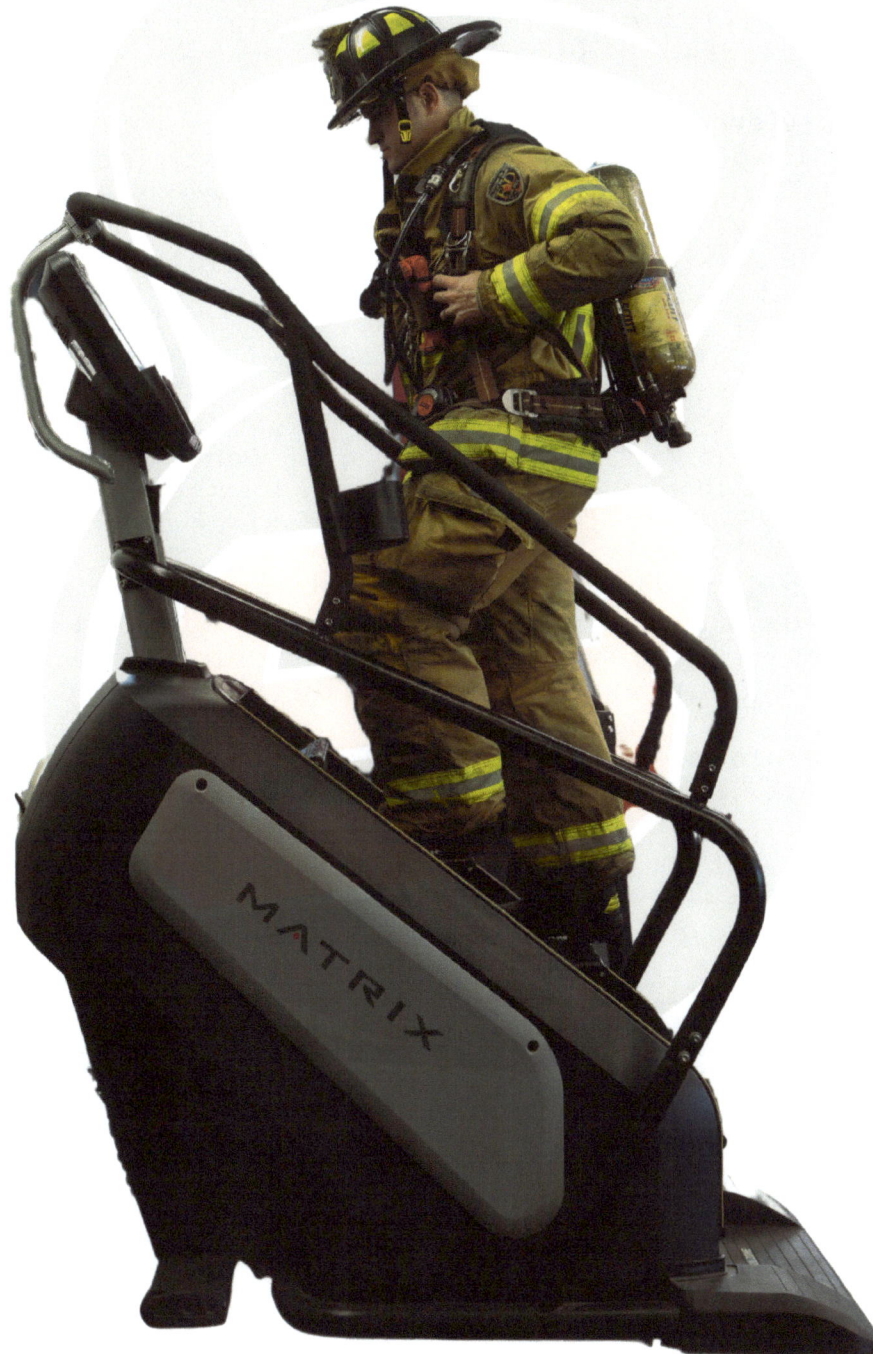

Stronger On Scene

"Progress, Not Perfection"

24 Day Stair Stepper Program

Welcome to the grind. This 24-day stair stepper program is built to push your limits, elevate your conditioning, and forge mental toughness through progressive overload and deliberate intensity. Whether your goal is tactical readiness, endurance dominance, or just pure grit, this program is designed to test and transform you.

Program Overview
This program is split into 5 progressive levels, each increasing in load and intensity. Each level is structured around weekly progressions in time and intensity. You'll climb, sweat, and grind through each level, building not just endurance, but the kind of willpower that lasts far beyond the machine.

Level Breakdown:
- **Level 1**: Bodyweight only –establish your base.
- **Level 2**: Add a 20lb vest –time to build some real work capacity.
- **Level 3**: Add a 40 lb vest –we're entering deep waters.
- **Level 4**: Add a 50 lb vest –strength & stamina fuse here.
- **Level 5**: Add a 75 lb vest –this is the proving ground.

Each week within a level will manipulate duration, step rate, and recovery periods to push your aerobic and muscular thresholds. Expect shorter, higher intensity sessions at the beginning of each level, building toward longer sustained efforts by the end.

Progression Protocol
To move up a level, you must complete at least 90% of the prescribed workouts for that level. If you fall short—good. That means the program is working. But don't skip ahead. Repeat the level until you hit that 90% threshold. This ensures not just physical readiness, but also the mental discipline this program demands.

Expectations & Mindset
This is not a casual cardio program. This is for people with lofty goals and relentless mindsets. You're going to sweat, fail, and question why you started. But if you commit, stay consistent, and respect the process, you'll come out harder, stronger, and more durable than ever before.

If you're ready to get after it, then let's climb.
Time to earn every step.

Stair Stepper
Level 1: No Weight

Day 1		
Time	**Steps/Min**	**Approx Level**
3 Min	42 s/m	Level 4
1 Min	54 s/m	Level 6
3 Min	60 s/m	Level 7

Day 2		
Time	**Steps/Min**	**Approx Level**
3 Min	42 s/m	Level 4
3 Min	60 s/m	Level 7
3 Min	42 s/m	Level 4
3 Min	60 s/m	Level 7

Day 3		
Time	**Steps/Min**	**Approx Level**
1 Min	42 s/m	Level 4
1 Min	54 s/m	Level 6
1 Min	60 s/m	Level 7
1 Min	72 s/m	Level 9
1 Min	83 s/m	Level 11
1 Min	42 s/m	Level 4
1 Min	72 s/m	Level 9
4 Min	42 s/m	Level 4

4 ROUNDS

Stair Stepper
Level 1: No Weight

Day 3		
Time	**Steps/Min**	**Approx Level**
2 Min	42 s/m	Level 4
4 Min	60 s/m	Level 7
4 Min	54 s/m	Level 6

Day 4		
Time	**Steps/Min**	**Approx Level**
15 Min	54 s/m	Level 6
This is more about stamina of simply staying on the machine and mentally digging in to accomplish the goal.		

Day 5		
Time	**Steps/Min**	**Approx Level**
1 Min	42 s/m	Level 4
2 Min	60 s/m	Level 7
1 Min	42 s/m	Level 4
2 Min	72 s/m	Level 9
1 Min	42 s/m	Level 4
3 Min	Rest	-
Complete 2 rounds of the above		

Stronger On Scene

Stair Stepper
Level 2: 20 lb vest

Day 6		
Time	**Steps/Min**	**Approx Level**
1 Min	60 s/m	Level 7
1 Min	Rest	-
Complete 7 Rounds		

Day 7		
Time	**Steps/Min**	**Approx Level**
2 Min	60 s/m	Level 7
2 Min	Rest	-
Complete 6 Rounds		

Day 8		
Time	**Steps/Min**	**Approx Level**
3 Min	60 s/m	Level 7
1:30 Min	Rest	-
Complete 5 Rounds		

Day 9		
Time	**Steps/Min**	**Approx Level**
10 Min	60 s/m	Level 7
Build confidence at this speed		

Stair Stepper
Level 3: 40 lb vest

Day 10		
Time	**Steps/Min**	**Approx Level**
:30	68-75	Level 8-10
:60	42 s/m	Level 4
Complete 7 Rounds		

Day 11		
Time	**Steps/Min**	**Approx Level**
:30	42 s/m	Level 4
:60	54 s/m	Level 6
:30	42 s/m	Level 4
:60	60 s/m	Level 7
:30	42 s/m	Level 4
:60	65 s/m	Level 8
:30	42 s/m	Level 4
3 Minute Rest Complete 2 Rounds		

Day 12		
Time	**Steps/Min**	**Approx Level**
:60	60 s/m	Level 7
:30	83 s/m	Level 11
:60	60 s/m	Level 7
:30	89 s/m	Level 12
:60	42 s/m	Level 4
2 Min	Rest	-
Complete two rounds of the above		

Stronger On Scene

Stair Stepper
Level 4: 50 lb vest

Day 13		
Time	**Steps/Min**	**Approx Level**
3 Min	60 s/m	Level 7
1:30 Min	Rest	-
Complete 3 Rounds		

Day 14		
Time	**Steps/Min**	**Approx Level**
:30	42 s/m	Level 4
:60	54 s/m	Level 6
:30	42 s/m	Level 4
:60	60 s/m	Level 7
:30	42 s/m	Level 4
:60	60 s/m	Level 7
:30	42 s/m	Level 4
3 Minute Rest Complete 2 Rounds		

Day 15		
Time	**Steps/Min**	**Approx Level**
15 Minutes		
S/M is your choice, only requirement is DO NOT GET OFF		
Build Mental Fortitude		

Stronger On Scene

Stair Stepper
Level 4: 50 lb vest

Day 16- PART 1		
Time	**Steps/Min**	**Approx Level**
:20	72-77 s/m	Level 9-10
:40	42 s/m	Level 4
Complete 4 Rounds		

Day 16- PART 2		
Time	**Steps/Min**	**Approx Level**
:20	80-85 s/m	Level 11
:40	42 s/m	Level 4
Complete 3 Rounds		

Day 17- PART 1		
Time	**Steps/Min**	**Approx Level**
:45	72-77 s/m	Level 9-10
:45	42 s/m	Level 4
Complete 4 Rounds		

Day 17- PART 2		
Time	**Steps/Min**	**Approx Level**
:45	83-89 s/m	Level 11-12
:45	42 s/m	Level 4
Complete 3 Rounds		

Day 18		
Time	**Steps/Min**	**Approx Level**
:60	60 s/m	Level 7
:90	42 s/m	Level 4
Complete 7 Rounds		

Stronger On Scene

Stair Stepper
Level 5: 75 lb vest

Day 19

Time	Steps/Min	Approx Level
1 Min	Any s/m	-
2 Min	Rest	-
Complete 5 Rounds		

Day 20

Time	Steps/Min	Approx Level
1:30	Any s/m	-
1:30	Rest	-
Complete 5 Rounds		

Day 21

Time	Steps/Min	Approx Level
2 Min	Any s/m	-
1 Min	Rest	-
Complete 5 Rounds		

Day 22

Time	Steps/Min	Approx Level
1 Min	60 s/m	Level 7
2 Min	42 s/m	Level 4
Complete 7 Rounds		

Day 23

Time	Steps/Min	Approx Level
2 Min	60 s/m	Level 7
2 Min	42 s/m	Level 4
Complete 5 Rounds		

Day 24

Time	Steps/Min	Approx Level
3 Min	60 s/m	Level 7
1 Min	42 s/m	Level 4
Complete 4 Rounds		

Day	Difficulty	Notes	✅	❌	Repeated
Day 1	Level 1				
Day 2	Level 1				
Day 3	Level 1				
Day 4	Level 1				
Day 5	Level 1				
Day 6	Level 2				
Day 7	Level 2				
Day 8	Level 2				
Day 9	Level 2				
Day 10	Level 3				
Day 11	Level 3				
Day 12	Level 3				
Day 13	Level 4				
Day 14	Level 4				
Day 15	Level 4				
Day 16	Level 4				
Day 17	Level 4				
Day 18	Level 4				
Day 19	Level 5				
Day 20	Level 5				
Day 21	Level 5				
Day 22	Level 5				
Day 23	Level 5				
Day 24	Level 5				

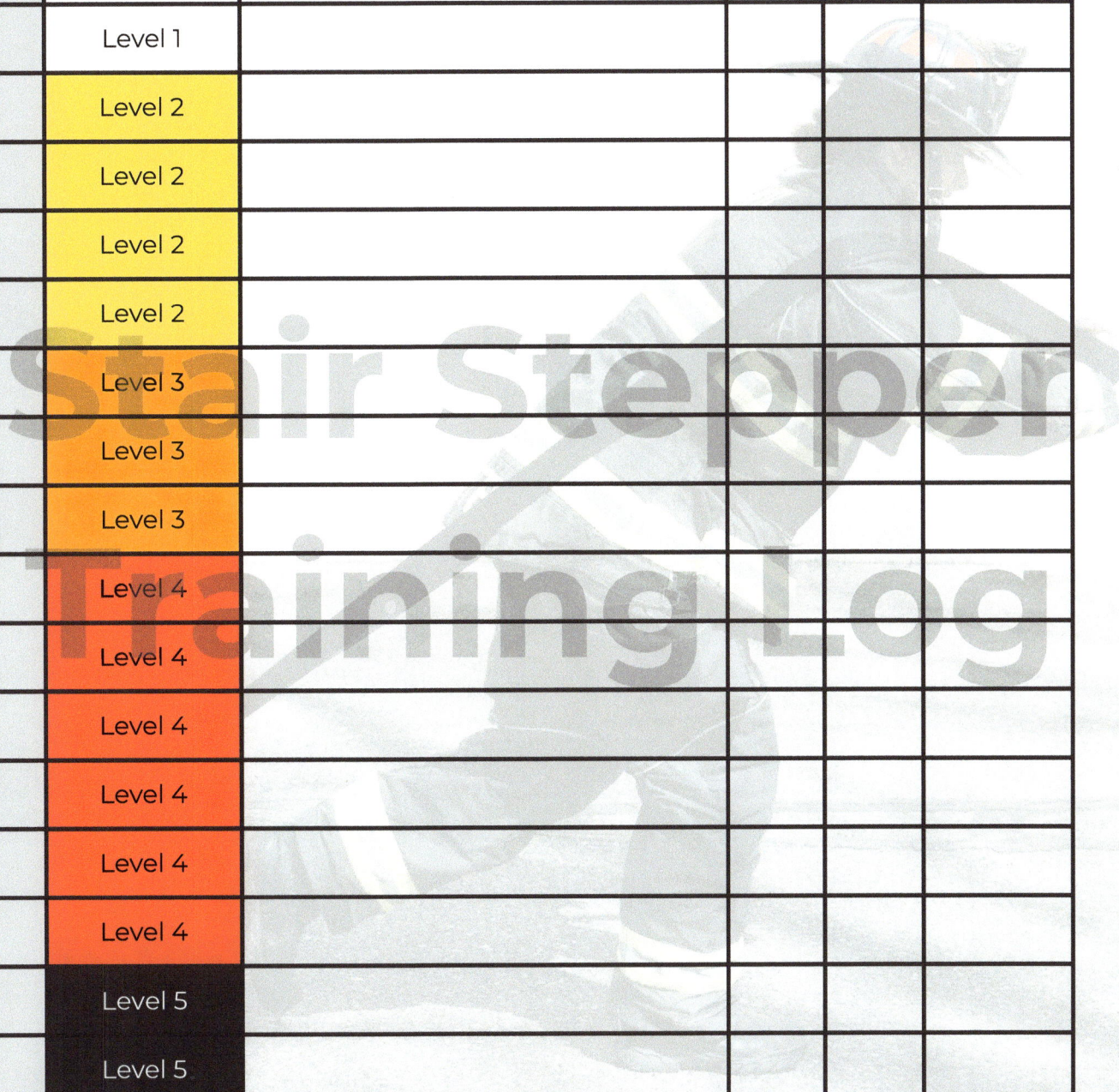

Stair Stepper Training Log

91

Day 1	On Shift-Off Shift-Before Shift

Notes

Rounds/Reps/Weights

Day 2	On Shift-Off Shift-Before Shift

Notes

Rounds/Reps/Weights

Day 3	On Shift-Off Shift-Before Shift

Notes

Rounds/Reps/Weights

Day 4	On Shift-Off Shift-Before Shift

Notes

Rounds/Reps/Weights

Day 5	On Shift-Off Shift-Before Shift

Notes

Rounds/Reps/Weights

Day 6	On Shift-Off Shift-Before Shift

Notes

Rounds/Reps/Weights

Day 7	On Shift-Off Shift-Before Shift

Notes

Rounds/Reps/Weights

Day 8	On Shift-Off Shift-Before Shift

Notes

Rounds/Reps/Weights

Day 9	On Shift-Off Shift-Before Shift

Notes

Rounds/Reps/Weights

Day 10	On Shift-Off Shift-Before Shift

Notes

Rounds/Reps/Weights

Day 11	On Shift-Off Shift-Before Shift

Notes

Rounds/Reps/Weights

Day 12	On Shift-Off Shift-Before Shift

Notes

Rounds/Reps/Weights

Day 13	On Shift-Off Shift-Before Shift

Notes

Rounds/Reps/Weights

Day 14	On Shift-Off Shift-Before Shift

Notes

Rounds/Reps/Weights

Day 15	On Shift-Off Shift-Before Shift

Notes

Rounds/Reps/Weights

Day 16	On Shift-Off Shift-Before Shift

Notes

Rounds/Reps/Weights

Day 17	On Shift-Off Shift-Before Shift

Notes

Rounds/Reps/Weights

Day 17	On Shift-Off Shift-Before Shift

Notes

Rounds/Reps/Weights

Day 18	On Shift-Off Shift-Before Shift

Notes

Rounds/Reps/Weights

Day 19	On Shift-Off Shift-Before Shift

Notes

Rounds/Reps/Weights

Day 20	On Shift-Off Shift-Before Shift

Notes

Rounds/Reps/Weights

Day 21	**On Shift-Off Shift-Before Shift**

Notes

Rounds/Reps/Weights

Day 22	**On Shift-Off Shift-Before Shift**

Notes

Rounds/Reps/Weights

Day 23	**On Shift-Off Shift-Before Shift**

Notes

Rounds/Reps/Weights

Day 24	**On Shift-Off Shift-Before Shift**

Notes

Rounds/Reps/Weights

Day 25	**On Shift-Off Shift-Before Shift**

Notes

Rounds/Reps/Weights

Day 26	**On Shift-Off Shift-Before Shift**

Notes

Rounds/Reps/Weights

Day 30	On Shift-Off Shift-Before Shift

Notes

Rounds/Reps/Weights

Day 31	On Shift-Off Shift-Before Shift

Notes

Rounds/Reps/Weights

Day 32	On Shift-Off Shift-Before Shift

Notes

Rounds/Reps/Weights

Day 33	On Shift-Off Shift-Before Shift

Notes

Rounds/Reps/Weights

Day 34	On Shift-Off Shift-Before Shift

Notes

Rounds/Reps/Weights

Day 35	On Shift-Off Shift-Before Shift

Notes

Rounds/Reps/Weights

Day 36	On Shift-Off Shift-Before Shift

Notes

Rounds/Reps/Weights

Day 37	On Shift-Off Shift-Before Shift

Notes

Rounds/Reps/Weights

Day 38	On Shift-Off Shift-Before Shift

Notes

Rounds/Reps/Weights

Day 39	**On Shift-Off Shift-Before Shift**

Notes

Rounds/Reps/Weights

Day 40	**On Shift-Off Shift-Before Shift**

Notes

Rounds/Reps/Weights

Day 41	**On Shift-Off Shift-Before Shift**

Notes

Rounds/Reps/Weights

Day 42	On Shift-Off Shift-Before Shift

Notes

Rounds/Reps/Weights

Day 43	On Shift-Off Shift-Before Shift

Notes

Rounds/Reps/Weights

Day 44	On Shift-Off Shift-Before Shift

Notes

Rounds/Reps/Weights

Day 45	**On Shift-Off Shift-Before Shift**

Notes

Rounds/Reps/Weights

Extra	**On Shift-Off Shift-Before Shift**

Notes

Rounds/Reps/Weights

Extra	**On Shift-Off Shift-Before Shift**

Notes

Rounds/Reps/Weights

www.ingramcontent.com/pod-product-compliance
Lightning Source LLC
Chambersburg PA
CBHW041420290326
41932CB00042B/36